THE RIDDLE IN THE MIRROR

A Journey in Search of Healing

JAYNI BLOCH

BALBOA.
PRESS
A DIVISION OF HAY HOUSE

Balboa Press books may be ordered through booksellers or by contacting:

Balboa Press
A Division of Hay House
1663 Liberty Drive
Bloomington, IN 47403
www.balboapress.com
1-(877) 407-4847

ISBN: 978-1-4525-5940-7 (sc)
ISBN: 978-1-4525-5941-4 (e)
ISBN: 978-1-4525-5942-1 (hc)

Library of Congress Control Number: 2012919279

Printed in the United States of America

Balboa Press rev. date: 11/19/2012

CONTENTS

List Of Illustrations

To my loving and supportive husband, Gerald, who is my inspiring partner in my healing journey and to my son, Anton, who is the continuation of this voyage.

"We find that the unconscious connects us to other people and to our entire environment; therefore when we focus a great deal of energy within the inner world, a parallel energy often arises in the people or situations around us. In this way, we can do healing through our inner work that we never could have done through external means."

—R. A. Johnson, *Inner Work*

You must understand the whole of life, not just one little part of it. That is why you must read, that is why you must look at the skies, that is why you must sing and dance, and write poems, and suffer, and understand, for all that is life."

—Jiddu Krishnamurti

INTRODUCTION

Contemplation is the ability to reflect on experiences. The mirror or any shiny reflective object, like the moon or a pool of water, symbolizes this ability. We see another dimension of experienced reality in the reflection. The formal reality of the visible world serves as such a reflector, a mirror that symbolizes a meaning beyond our human mind's interpretation of what we experience. In this way we then connect to the true story of an eternal dimension of life and not the subjective dimension only. This reflected dimension is truer in a spiritual sense because it gives us perspective on a bigger universal reality of our being's evolution as a part of a bigger whole.

A mirror is the symbol of imagination and consciousness. Dreams, symbols, and synchronicities resemble the reflective qualities of a mirror and put us in touch with memories, the unconscious, and the universal aspect of life. *The Riddle in the Mirror* deals with our connection with the universal principles of life, using knowledge of archetypal symbolism to understand how our life events, dreams, and synchronicities inform us about our healing processes. Such contemplation opens our awareness to the collective reality that extends our rational thought and ego-only awareness, so that we can find meaning in our challenges.

When we reflect on life and our experience as a metaphor that indicates our current position on a dynamic map of evolution, our latent inner spiritual side awakes. Before this awakening, our lives are completely involved with material ambitions where our past conditioning by family and society dictates our behavior and motives by fear and need. Our spiritual sides are unconscious because of our conditioning to perceive only our subjective impressions. Our spiritual sides try to reach us by communicating through our physical symptoms and uncomfortable emotional sensations. It is amazing how much we occupy ourselves with cognitive thoughts and ideas that shut down our inner voice with its ability to illuminate deeper meaning. The process of self-reflection is a vital one for finding our true self, life purpose, and destiny. Finding our inner voice is tricky because of the determination of our ego structure that revels in maintaining its socialized identity. While any extreme personal circumstance can trigger awareness of our spiritual dimension, the favorable times for our self-reflective ability seem to occur as an "awakening" around the age of twenty-eight to thirty-five and again around the age of fifty-five to fifty-six. We can however intentionally seek our awareness of our deeper self through practicing self-contemplation. Once we know how to reflect on our lives, self-reflection becomes a healing tool. We find direction and purpose once we connect to the truth of our being by reflecting on the archetypal symbolism of experience.

Every day, I experience the astonishing reality of how the reflection on the symbolism of events brings the truth to our attention in powerful ways. We often block our ability to understand true meaning by our clever ability to use rationalizations and defense mechanisms in dealing with emotional unhappiness. Our personality usually circles a dilemma from all the possible cognitive angles and comes to some great theory to explain the happening. We can even formulate possible solutions for the issue, but most of the time there is no sensation of resolution. A "click", the sensation of resolve, happens when our reason connects to a deeper soul truth. Life becomes that mirror in which we access the truths of our soul's need to heal when we look at life from a symbolic angle. To do this, we need an understanding of the collective and archetypal principles of healing and spiritual growth.

Our experience of the visible and cognitive world reflects a universe of spiritual truth beyond the visible and cognitive world. Usually, the arrangement of symbolism in experiences or metaphors in dreams and circumstances opens a collective perspective that illuminates the logical information and provides answers to questions that our mind struggles to solve. Before the insight, which feels like a click our emotional challenges usually feel remote, as if outside circumstances are responsible for making mistakes that cause our misery and suffering.

We even blame ourselves for our circumstances instead of contemplating deeper growth challenges. There is no mistake as far as the unconscious goes. Our challenging experiences bring us awareness of our hidden wounds, which we would otherwise not detect. When our logic and our collective side agree with a solution or understanding, the click happens in our sensory body. The illuminating insight strikes with tremendous relief, despite its painful truth. Everything makes sense, and the true therapy can begin because the ego has no defense against the truth. Rationalization is redundant when we know what we need to do to heal.

Digging through the defense mechanisms to our soul's truth and the meaning of the challenges we face is no easy task. To find our true self, purpose, and destiny, we realize that all challenges serve as indicators for the truth that will set us free from the reparative ambush of conflict and life's emotional discomforts.

Challenges are the riddles to our rational selves. These riddles are life's mirror. *The Riddle in the Mirror* will help you look into the mirror of your life with the intention to perceive the universal symbolism that clarifies the true meaning of your struggles for the purpose of your growth and healing. Sometimes, the meaning in the struggle has nothing to do with what we rationally think of as practical solutions. Our soul's truth surprises us with its obvious simplicity, yet our reason resists this knowing with all its might. Our soul's truth is always unique to us; it does not necessarily apply to everyone, and brings forward a deeper reality about our human wounds that we usually try to hide from others and ourselves.

Rational analysis and practical problem-solving still apply, but they do not stand on their own. We cannot ignore the underlying shifts in attitude we need to adopt in order to complete our responsibility to emotional growth and spiritual evolution through completing our healing processes. The challenge to change relates directly to our conscious participation in personal spiritual growth and development. Our personal participation supports all of life's development. This is the only way we start to change and heal humanity.

The Riddle in the Mirror is partly a memoir that comes as the result of living the healing process through self-reflection on my own life experiences and observing and learned from other healers and therapists as well as my clients in my counseling practice over thirty years. This book demonstrates how we identify the healing opportunities in the challenges we encounter. Although personal, our challenges are part of a collective journey of healing. Our personal challenges are never isolated from our familial, cultural, or ancestral histories. These historical roots affect our views, beliefs, and behavior in dealing with life.

The Riddle in the Mirror tells the story of how my own search for healing and understanding started during times of personal crisis, how I found it related to my cultural history, and how these influences ignited a personal healing journey. I observed how my socially conditioned ideas affected my internal dialogue and consequently how I perceive and respond to life. Once I started asking transpersonal questions because of my emotional pain, I started experiencing events that empirical psychology could not explain. These circumstances prompted me to explore healing from the inside out and from the outside in, searching beyond the realm of pure science as we know it today. This awareness gave me the courage to change.

I share my personal observations, investigations, experiences, and findings with you to inspire you on your own healing journey. This book is not an academic book but a personal perspective that was born from experience, observation, contemplation. I hope to inspire you in your search for your own answers to your life's questions. Take from this book what you feel is appropriate and practical for your own life. Heal by listening to your own true inner guidance. Distinguish between your truth and the fabrication that your ego or social conditioning tells you to believe.

The Riddle in the Mirror describes a conceptual model of the purpose and function of our ego-based personality. This model supports us with a diagram that clarifies our understanding of how our ego functions and how to integrate our spiritual side with our ego-side. Our ego is an essential mechanism in our personality, but living life on its own abilities robs us of being whole. When our ego and all its aspects connect to the divine aspect of our psyche, we develop our true self. I encountered many master-mentors in person and through books. This model came about as a composite of my own understanding and those from their teachings. My heartfelt appreciation goes to all the brilliant teachers, thinkers, and healers who have opened the path to healing and affected my life significantly.

As a whole, our divine side consists of a collection of archetypal qualities. Our divine side manifests itself in the ego-personality through a consciousness of the fact that the divine already exists within us. As we discover these faces of God in us, through healing our wounds that challenge us, we become whole selves again. The revolutionary realization of *The Riddle in the Mirror* is about healing the disconnected parts of us as individuals but also of how we belong together as humanity.

These faces of God are universal archetypes, operating as one whole and which exist in all of life. They express themselves in the unfolding creative life force of the universe as co-operating qualities. We become aware of these qualities as they manifest as time-sensitive processes in our physical experiences and circumstances as developmental phases adding conscious understanding one upon another like building blocks until we grasp wholeness. We become conscious of these qualities though recognizing the symbolic themes in our experiences. Instead of our socialized conditioning, these new insights and awareness's of the archetypal symbolism in events, guides our adjustments in our choices of behaviors so that we participate in growth and healing. Each of us carries the parts of the whole as individuals and as cultural units. Life itself reflects back to us who we are.

Human development, as reflected by history, also unfolds according to these archetypal patterns and qualities. We observe the methodical unfolding of the archetypal lessons that awaken our divine qualities by understanding the language of archetypal symbolism and the collective unconscious. When disconnected from our divine side, our personalities identifies with the interpretations that our ego invents about our experiences. The story our ego tells us usually trap us in repetitive conflict cycles which are reactive fear based behavior that perpetuate our wounds and the wounding of each other and the earth. Each challenge that we face becomes a healing phase where our personalities have an opportunity to move out of its repetitive defensive patterns toward true healing and growth.

The divine qualities in the traits that our egos reveal through our personalities stay latent until we discover them by looking beyond the mundane into the mirror of collective symbolism. Symbolism guides our egos to connect with soul and therefore approach challenges more objectively. The almost tedious processes of life teach us through painful experiences to connect with all that we are instead of the one-sided perspective of our ego alone. Symbolism connects us with archetypal "messages" that wake us up to wholeness. It is our soul's contribution to rational understanding and meaning of events. Our soul speaks through the symbolism in our physical bodies, our dreams and synchronistic circumstances. Through conscious living, we have an opportunity to attune ourselves to these archetypal processes and thus connect with the divine aspect of our nature in a healing process that results in wholeness. Enjoy the journey.

CHAPTER 1

Lineage

History Is Important

History unmistakably expresses the progression of humankind's evolution in every regard: emotionally, physically, socially, intellectually, and spiritually. Everyone has a personal and a family history. Our cultural past plays a major role in our personal psychological health and formulation of a worldview. The way we move through life depends on the cultural narrative of our time. We absorb the themes of our time like sponges in the same way we do family attitudes.

Every generation has its own stories. As long as we are unconscious of them, we do not have a choice about how their themes and conflicts affect us. These themes inevitably ignite psychological wounds from time to time in unexpected ways. Even if we are conscious of these themes, we may still struggle to integrate them with an objective perspective, especially when atrocities or hardships taint our history. This is why most of us struggle with the question of how to heal ourselves, especially when our history reappears in wounding or shaming memories.

Our personalities have a tendency to discard our history. We rationalize it, keep on suffering it, ignore it, or compensate for it. Our society reiterates the wounds of history, reinforcing blame and a sense of victimhood, by relaying specific biased ideas in narratives that influence our thoughts. These ideas and beliefs, which we repeat in our minds and stories, bond us to their pain. It is difficult to know how to heal the wounding events of life. It can be a lifelong process for individuals to heal personal and generational wounds, and it takes even longer for cultures to heal. When communities struggle with the consequences of cultural history, the wounds are carried over from generation to generation.

Our soul-spirit urgently presses a need in us to heal by exposing us to crises. Its message about how to change ourselves lies in the symbolism of the crisis on condition that we interpret this symbolism with the right faculty. Our ego and rational mind can lead us astray when it comes to symbolism. Symbolism is found in the themes of our wounds. The stories of our culture, the stories of our families, and our personal story relate and carry some commonality. We suffer generational themes in personal ways. Therefore even if we think we are unattached to our history we notice that cultural and familial stories narrate our personal struggles. Our wounds are part of our human destiny and they connect us to archetypal themes that urge our development beyond our current perspective; as a persona and as humanity. By participating in our personal healing, we participate with the creative universe in changing personal as well as collective patterns of human consciousness and behavior. I consider the personal healing process intimately intertwined with cultural healing.

My healing journey began in South Africa where I started life. I was born into an atmosphere of conflict which became the instigator of my search for peace. It is apparent when reading the history of South Africa that conflict, hostility, and rivalry—especially in the form of war—were rampant over long periods between the different groups of people who occupied and shared the land. Growing up in this atmosphere of open— and sometimes denied—conflict and bias was psychologically traumatic. Especially covert conflict confused my child-mind. There was a continuous underlying psychological battle for the upper hand, prejudice and control, while people pretended to tolerated each other. My homeland was a warring place. The many cultural groups that formed the peoples of South Africa were all in conflict with each other.

Children have a natural ability to love and reach out to each other without bias. They start life free from prejudice until their mentors' attitudes teach them differently. Children know what the adults around them think and feel without knowing that they know, and they absorb these judgments. Children unknowingly take on the biases of the adults. A sense of suffering encourages our primal survival instincts when we feed resentments and ideas about injustices done to us. These kinds of biases can easily perpetuate from generation to generation. The emotional atmosphere in South Africa during my childhood was one such rivalry; each cultural group was trying to protect its own—even if it was to the disadvantage of others. As I matured I became more conscious of the intensity of cultural conflict in my country. I longed for a peaceful, unbiased, and loving community and even though I did not want any part of that conflict, my psyche carried the wounds of my history unconsciously.

When everyone tries to conquer who they perceive as their enemies in a diverse but extreme prejudice and intolerant community, we are tempted to harm each other for our own benefit and staying power instead of supporting each other to grow and heal. This attitude enhances and propagates eternal human conflict against all that are different from you. These same conflicting attitudes in politics replicate among children in schools, communities, and families. When no one knows any better, no one knows how to change this vicious cycle.

Friction can stimulate creativity and innovation and is therefore potentially liberating, but can also be incredibly destructive. Conflict can lead us to shift our past or current point of view or keep us adamant about convictions. Conflict has us fear losing our standing, convictions, or values. Everyone on earth has experienced to one degree or another creative as well as destructive times because of the consequences of conflict. The leaders of our time guide the direction of the consequence of conflict to be helpful or hurtful in communities. We need principled parents and cultural leaders to guide society not leaders that influence destruction of relationships. True leaders help us learn to listen to one another's perspectives without bias so that we can reach a peaceful understanding of each other. Our wise, visionary leaders—men and women who lead from a place outside of self-interest—can channel the sparks that conflict creates toward cooperation instead of war and competition. True leaders encourage healthy relationships among all people to benefit everyone, not just combating ones. These kinds of leaders are rare. Nelson Mandela and F. W. de Klerk are two such leaders.

If we want to grow and evolve, we all need to heal the past and move beyond the repetitive nature of holding regrets, resentments, wounds, and vengeful attitudes. Justifying our anger because of past atrocities is obsolete. Let us step into each other's worlds with compassion and let go of our misleading perspectives. It is difficult to be neutral when we are emotionally affected, and this is where we need true social and personal leaders to support and guide us in a healing process with practical spiritual principles.

The conflicting attitudes among various cultural groups during my upbringing mirror the many coexisting inner points of view that we find in our individual psyches. The world outside us reflects the world inside us and the other way round. There are many parts, some of which we are unconscious of, that completes us. Some of these parts compete with others for a position of power within our personalities. Our soul battles for wholeness, so that all of the parts of our personality co-operatively unite in our psyche. Our personalities on the other hand love to rule our being with an ego state or two. This results in us not realizing that we are far more than the sum of the parts. Humanity is destined to cooperate spiritually, but our personalities are trained to look out for their own needs and therefore ignore the soul's calling in experiences of unhappiness. Without the unease of external conflict that brings awareness of the internal battles between the parts of our egos, the urge to change would not happen. Without discomfort, there is no spark toward growth or need to discover solutions within one's self and between societies and cultures. Our personal healing always ripples out toward humanity.

People all over the world live in physical, emotional, and spiritual exile, needing to heal relationships, families, cultures, or countries. Different people and cultures share universal patterns in their personal lives that connect us all as one human family. In the search for healing, we all share the longing to find "home," a place of belonging where we all give each other acceptance, respect, and nurturing support. When we find "home" within ourselves, humanity is a step closer to finding peace with each other. Our individual stories are not identical—just as our cultural stories are not—but our experiences bind us in a common evolutionary challenge. We grow through the healing process as individuals, cultures, and humankind as a whole.

CHAPTER 2

Climbing the Mountain

The weight of fear crushes our connection to the meaning of life because it triggers survival instincts that taint human perception. Struck with fear and sadness or greed and desire when met with challenges, we sever ourselves from our ability to connect to our spiritual insight for guidance. Initially challenges are riddles to our mind as we struggle to find answers, but from the perspective of our spirit, every painful experience clearly reveals the way to heal.

The healing process is like climbing a mountain. In meditation or during sleep, ask God-in-you what you should make of the burdens you carry. A drop-of-God exists inside everyone. In the silence of this symbolic walk up the mountain, your God-self opens insight like an eye at the center of your being. Your heart starts to glow with new vision and useful perspectives. You see your difficulties are in reality the seeds that stir transformation in you. Communicate with your inner God-side and walk the mountain of contemplation in silence, listening and observing. This silence is a symbolic place between heaven and earth where all opposites disappear. Light and dark unite; sorrow and joy merge. Heaven grows on earth, and earth expresses heaven in its growth.

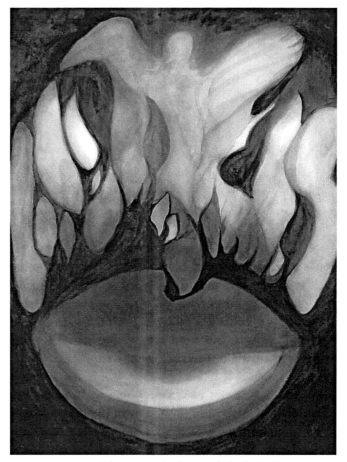

Inner Sight. Watercolor by Jayni Bloch, 2004

How It All Started

I was born during the peak of apartheid in Johannesburg, South Africa. Trade restrictions isolated our connection with the rest of the world. Global and local news was controlled. A fundamental divide existed, most obviously between black and white people in South Africa, but multiple other divides immersed the country. After the Boer War, the white population split its alliance between Afrikaans and English-speaking peoples. Most English-speaking people had alliances to the British who were involved in a massacre of the Boers, (mostly Afrikaans women and children who were put in concentration camps during the war).

The Afrikaans people carried much resentment against this carnage, which in turn fueled more animosity between them and the English-speaking groups. I first experienced awareness of group hostility at school when the children severely bullied each other. They based their differences on language.

South Africa is home to many different ethnic groups, as well as many immigrant cultures. Of the 45 million South Africans, there are nearly 31 million blacks, 5 million whites, 3 million colored (mixed race), and 1 million Indians. At the time of this writing, the population density is 32.9 people per km². There are four major ethnic groups among the black population, namely Nguni, Sotho, Shangaan-Tsonga, and Venda. The Zulu and Xhosa (two subgroups of the Nguni) are the largest of numerous subgroups. The majority of the white population is of Afrikaans descent (60 percent), with many of the remaining 40 percent being of British descent. Most of the colored population lives in the Northern and Western Cape provinces, while most of the Indian population lives in KwaZulu Natal.

The Afrikaner population is concentrated in the Gauteng and Free State provinces, and the English population resides in the Western and Eastern Cape and KwaZulu Natal. There are eleven official languages in South Africa: English, Afrikaans, Ndebele, Sepedi, Xhosa, Venda, Tswana, Southern Sotho, Zulu, Swazi, and Tsonga.

From 1652 until 1835, migrant and refugee Calvinist Protestants—primarily from France, the Netherlands, Germany, Scotland, and elsewhere in Europe—came to South Africa, following the example of the French Huguenots in the early 1600s. Their persecution lasted for a hundred years after the revocation of the Edict of Nantes. There was also an infusion of Indian and Malaysian people brought to South Africa to help farm the land in the 1600s.

By the end of the eighteenth century, these persecuted Europeans no longer identified themselves as such, but rather as Afrikaners. The new integrated culture called the Afrikaners assimilated from many of the original immigrants as well as local people. The Afrikaners became a group of explorers who wanted freedom to farm and serve their religion with freedom. They developed a new indigenous language, called Afrikaans which had roots in all their combined original European languages. Their Calvinist religion (*Nederduits Gereformeerde Kerk*) as well as their new language bound them together. Any threat to their newfound freedom instilled an oppressive collective fear. Paradoxically, the very religion that brought these diverse people together later underlies the divide of the country of South Africa.

Ten years after the Anglo-Boer War, the Afrikaners negotiated a home-rule arrangement in the four British colonies, and firmly established themselves as the ruling minority in South Africa. Their policies became one of exclusive control, called apartheid. After long struggles between the cultural groups over many years, F. W. de Klerk recognized the absurdity of apartheid and negotiated freeing Nelson Mandela from prison where he played a major role with his vision of freedom for all cultural groups in South Africa. The abolishment of apartheid announced a new era in the history of South Africa.

Afrikaner Calvinism, according to theory, is a unique cultural development that combined the Calvinist religion with the political aspirations of the white Afrikaans-speaking people of South Africa. Consciously and unconsciously, they reinforced a dictatorial and authoritarian social climate that controlled the nation's thoughts, under the illusion of protecting the Afrikaners from oppressive forces. The Afrikaners, compelled by loyalty to each other, the Church, and the State, protected their identity against oppression by the British, especially after the Boer War. The Afrikaner people's paranoia of suppression resulted in isolating themselves culturally.

The Afrikaner government managed a censorship program that prevented contact with the rest of the world. The government of South Africa monitored all information available to its citizens by manipulating information in all media. Blinkered and isolated, the people of South Africa, especially the Afrikaners, understood and interpreted events through a shroud of delusion. Government and church indoctrination promoted fearful survival instincts in this small group of white people. The rest of the cultural groups living in South Africa fractured into categories where language, religion, and color would define and distinguish them. All the groups mistrusted each other. Every person's color and language immediately indicated their particular class. Assumptions discounted all individual beliefs and sentiments. Your language and color immediately labeled you no matter what your individual ideas, which was never asked only assumed.

Survival of the fittest and caring for your own kind ruled the everyday ambience. Every cultural group felt righteous and victimized at the same time. Consciously, everyone overtly denied mistrusting each other, but conflict and discrimination were distinct.

This discriminatory atmosphere severely distressed me as a child. It was confusing to observe people treat others without respect or fairness while the Church and State constantly preached humanistic values. Groups kept fracturing from each other. All the cultural groups treated each other with bias. It embarrassed and confused me, so I did not allow myself to identify with any one group. I felt lost without a sense of belonging. I felt a part of everyone, yet no-one. At times, I tried hard to belong but always felt uncomfortable. My ideas of union were often judged. An internal sense of ideological detachment grew stronger and left me emotionally alienated. I did not belong yet I was part of a judgmental culture who excluded others. These were the only people I knew and I was an outcast if they knew how I felt inside.

The motto on the South African coat of arms was "Unity is Strength." I really liked the idea of unity and longed for it to be a reality, but people's behavior toward each other was at odds with that concept. Even the verbal proclamation of good principles and intentions only applied within a cohesive group and never towards people outside of one's own group. I very soon learned that the execution of principles and ideas often contradicted the verbal declaration of them. Maybe a culture adopts a motto that their souls recognize as the one they most need to learn. Maybe individuals are part of a culture with a motto that as individuals we need to understand and act on, not only unwittingly accept. Unquestionably, I wanted to learn about the true nature of unity grown from diversity.

This young new Afrikaner culture was initially a neglected group of people whom the British considered inferior. Sprouting from persecuted European immigrants, the Afrikaner people had no financial or educational status that gave them prestige in the eyes of the British who valued wealth and education. Afrikaans was a brand-new language that unfolded creatively from various diverse European and African languages because of the people's need to communicate with each other. Haunted by a history of persecution, they believed they had to protect their young language, new culture, and newfound freedom they desperately awaited.

Despite their exceptional creativity and productivity, the Afrikaner leaders turned into oppressors once they came in power. They served their own exclusivity. Though their motives may be honorable in the light of their wounds, they resembled the very enemy they resented by excluding the rest of the country's peoples.

Our psyches carry our so-called enemy inside ourselves even though we perceive this enemy as someone on the outside. Carl Gustav Jung described this kind of projection as our *shadow* nature. A conflict cycle links victims and perpetrators intimately through a shared wound, which makes our enemies part of our wound and therefore part of our healing. I believe that all the children of this time, no matter what culture or color, suffer deep wounds that link us to a healing process, if only we could see that. Cultural wounds inform us about our constructive and destructive actions and reactions to life during every era of human existence. Our cultural wounds continue from generation to generation until they are healed by individuals. Consciousness about our fears, defensiveness and puzzlement about who we truly are helps us stop repeating inflicting wounds on each other.

I grew up in Mondeor, a small town situated eleven kilometers south of Johannesburg where I was born. Our home rested in the center of a natural basin surrounded by *randjies.* The Bloubosspruit River ran its curves through the center of town. Columbine Avenue was the main road that cut a path through the center of Mondeor and connected roads to Johannesburg from opposite directions. It was significant to me to learn that Columbine was a Latin word for dove, the symbol of peace. This fact made me feel good to live there and always reminded me of what I stood for. To me, Mondeor was the most beautiful place on earth because of its proximity to nature. I imagined that the hills around Mondeor folded a magical circle around us. A few homes thinly spread across the valley in this new development that bordered on 615 hectares of natural fields and hills, filled with 150 species of birds and 650 indigenous plants and trees. This wildlife terrain adjacent Mondeor was proclaimed a nature reserve, called Klipriviersberg, in 1984. The area, my childhood playground, has a rich archeological history that dates back to the Stone Age, 250,000 years ago. There are ancient stone circles and the remains of dwellings as well as many artifacts of that time.

Just beyond the periphery, other southern Johannesburg suburbs contrasted with green peaceful Mondeor, with dusty yellow fabricated hills constructed from the residue of gold mining dust. The discovery of gold in 1886 resulted in the appearance of many of these mine-dumps dotted around the southern side of Johannesburg. The affluent north of the city had fewer visible dumps. Johannesburg snobbishly divided people into the wealthy northerners and poor southerners. Rich and poor was added to all the other divisions in South Africa.

Fine gold dust filled the Transvaal air during dry windy seasons. Life in Johannesburg was clouded in gold dust that constantly inflamed my eyes. I saw a dusty reality perceived through a veil of golden naiveté that hurt with its unfulfilled idealism. Wishing to find truth and authenticity, I became lost in dreams. My imagination provided a peaceful and happy life up to the point when I could not maintain the illusion.

My child-mind wanted to extinguish all visible adversity and ugliness that was so painful to bear. Escape is a crucial defense against hardship and conflict. Living on the edge of humanity, not quite belonging, I fantasized about harmony between all people and the beauty of creation that I found in nature. How did I belong in such a strange and uncomfortable world? I searched for hope and new possibilities in fantasy, but reality caught up with my escape.

School introduced me to society where I immediately felt robbed of all innocence. It was time for me to wake up from a sleep. All my trust in authority shattered when my first teacher humiliated me publicly by ridiculing my father's occupation. I felt deeply disrespected. The teacher's bias did not match her proclaimed moral stance. People act out their biases without awareness despite their declared moral intentions. Judgment and distrust made it unsafe to show anyone who I truly was. It was crucial to hide my soul.

It was dangerous to trust my own judgment because everyone liked this teacher. She had status in our society and knew all the important people like the doctors and the lawyers. I recognized my own undercover judgment of her and society because of this experience. I made myself feel wrong because *they* must be right. *How can I be the only one who feels the injustice?* I had to do things the way others wanted—or they might exclude me. I did not dare reveal my feelings or thoughts. My inconsistent environment expected conformity and loyalty from me. Too scared to be spontaneous, I shut myself away. An incoherent, biased society would not accept me, I thought, because I felt and thought so different from them. I do not honor the same values they did. I did not come from a family who had money, education, any particular status, or political power. How was I ever to belong?

My personal life reflected the wounds of my cultural heritage. Somehow, I carried the wounds of my time, reflected in my culture, in a personal way, so I could become aware of how to heal this.

I wondered how I can find and identify truth. How could I measure the reliability of information and knowledge? There was no one to talk to or guide me. Always keeping an open mind, I constantly checked to verify my ideas, ready to adjust my views from what I thought the truth might be at any particular time to the newfound awareness I might discover. It felt as if truth unfolded as my experience and awareness grew. I focused intensely on non-verbal cues to find new understanding. I could only trust truth that came from internal questioning and truth that came from others who proved their integrity. People with true integrity make one feel seen and understood. Only value the opinions of those who truly recognize you. Truth reveals itself in one's subtle observations of our intuitive senses. Attune yourself to the wordless, to how you feel in the company of people. Their authentic attitude reveals an ability to connect. Look at their faces, their eyes, and their posture. A person's considerate behavior communicates their integrity non-verbally much more powerfully than their words do. Verbal information alone is often misguiding and can belie hidden intentions. Our first impressions of visible reality never tell the full story, but our first intuitive impressions are often more powerful clues of truth.

Half the population in Mondeor spoke English, and the other half spoke Afrikaans. There was one school. Separate classrooms divided the children according to language, but tension raged between English and Afrikaans children. Derogative name-calling and unrestrained physical bullying sustained an unpleasant divide amongst children each day in the schoolyard.

Disturbed by the constant fighting at school, I asked my mother why Afrikaans and English people were so nasty to each other. She told me about the Boer War. I questioned the existence of war and was astonished to learn that it had ended a long time ago. Why then does the animosity continue between children of the adults who fought the war even though there was supposed to be peace? (The Second Boer War lasted from October 11, 1899 until May 31, 1902, between the British Empire and the two independent Boer republics, the Transvaal Republic and the Orange Free State.) It seemed that war continued in the minds of innocent children who still carried the unresolved wounds of their parents and ancestors. Why do children, who are not born prejudiced, still hold warlike attitudes from the past? I remembered my experience with the teacher who demonstrated her hurtful bias toward me without realizing the consequences of her behavior. Perhaps parents and adults perpetuate antagonism and prejudice in children when they do not heal themselves.

The ongoing conflict between groups of people who lived in the same town and shared the same school building was excruciatingly painful, but I lived as if everything was fine. It felt as if the unresolved bitterness and contempt people hold breeds more of the same and amplifies the vicious cycle. South Africa was a place of self-survival and everyone took care of only their own. Everyone tried to protect his or her singular identity as they belonged to a particular group. But there was no respect or acknowledgement of others. The lack of cooperation, respect, and integration disturbed me deeply.

I was horrified when my school announced a rule that forbade friendships between Afrikaans- and English-speaking kids. My best friend, Elaine, was English! Lucky for us both, our mothers encouraged us to continue our friendship, even if it meant that we did so after school. It was liberating to break the rules. We knew to disallow our friendship was wrong. I found the courage to "disobey." The ban strengthened our friendship which lasted for many years. But the threat of rejection from my culture, for doing what others did not, continued to haunt me.

More disturbing moral discrepancies were revealed as I engaged with the church community. Although they promoted love and acceptance of our neighbors, contact with people of other faiths or languages was unacceptable. It seemed hypocritical to preach love without applying it to all people even if they were of different faith. Having more confidence at the age of twelve and a distinct sense of morality, I naively confronted the preacher with this incongruity. The fierce disapproving expression on his face suggested that I had broken a cultural taboo, which instantly felt like a hostile rejection. I knew I was teetering on the edge of emotional denunciation from my community. A renewed sense of not fitting in overwhelmed me.

The Afrikaners were encouraged to educate themselves and to honor their language and religion. Regard for the authorities that oversaw all was fortified. The arts and, most of all, loyalty were encouraged. Thinking for oneself and questioning the status quo were discouraged when it came to religion and government. This authoritarian attitude suppressed my spontaneity. An unexpressed rule determined that emotional excommunication resulted if one did not accept, express, and practice the obligatory beliefs of the culture.

Education during that time excluded the contemplation of different points of view. Teachers, political leaders, and religious authorities reinforced cultural loyalty. Emotional ceremonies served as constant reminders of the Boer War atrocities that encouraged allegiance to protect our culture. Memories of the carnage toward the Afrikaner women and children during that war increased the fear of an "enemy" invasion that could rob or desecrate our identity, language, and land. Their sense of victimhood reinforced their efforts to segregate and educate themselves in an attempt to protect the Afrikaner identity. This defensive reaction is a normal human response to victimization. In order to moderate threats to one's identity and power, separating people into groups instilled a false guarantee of safety. This strategy, whether conscious or unconscious, perpetuated hatred and animosity through fear, resentment, and revenge. We all carry the wounds suffered by our ancestors. How do we learn from history without perpetuating hate? We suffer the undercurrents of cultural and ancestral wounds when our teachers and healers do not openly speak about these and guide us to heal. Our human tendency is to indulge in our emotional suffering instead of healing it. Suffering reinforces cultural identity and keeps us locked in our wounds. Contemplating our experiences and gathering the right information helps us process our wounds and heal.

Carl Gustav Jung talked about the collective unconscious when he described how our history influences our development that is dependent on our ancestral past.

> In so far as no man is born totally new, but continually repeats the stage of development last reached by the species, he contains unconsciously, as an *a priori* (known without experience) datum (information), the entire psychic structure developed both upwards and downwards by his ancestors in the course of the ages. That is what gives the unconscious its characteristic "historical" aspect, but it is at the same time the *sine qua non* (outcome) for shaping the future.

The hostilities between the Afrikaans- and English-speaking people were only the start of my discovery of complex tribalism in my country. I learned that the entire black population lived separately from white suburbs and that there were many tribes who lived with animosity toward each other. Why was there so much tension among different groups of people and religions? Why did authorities, church, schools, and government try to keep people separate? Does this not feed animosity instead of heal it? Open discussion about these issues was not encouraged. I suspected the conflict between people existed because they felt threatened about the survival of their group identities. The existence of these conflicts seeded an aspiration for harmony and integration. I believe humanity cannot operate outside of unity. Despite pushing each other into unacceptable categories and fighting for positions of power over each other, every identifiable group is just as necessary to the whole of humanity as the number of atoms in a molecule. We all belong together and have something to contribute and learn from each other.

The incentive to improve, and better the circumstances and status for the Afrikaner nation, became an unhealthy obsession under the leadership of the apartheid government. The government's approach to healing our culture's deep scar of feeling oppressed created a need to control, thus leading them to control others. This led to deceiving the very culture they wanted to protect. Oppressing others for the sake of uplifting oneself is a form of deception that haunts and fractures everyone involved. All groups tend to compete for their own advantages and those who have leadership and power over others can take advantage of this sentiment. Let us learn from history and not repeat the mistakes. This attitude of self-promotion is a human tendency, wherever it happens, but it is also a spiritual flaw that demonstrates a consequential destruction throughout the history of humankind. Celebrating victory in the face of another's adversity is an animalistic instinct that stems from survival fear. We start our human life with this fear and need to grow beyond it. Therefore, if we are ever to advance and become "whole," we need to overturn the attitude of self-centeredness in favor of an attitude of compassion. Are we emotionally and spiritually mature enough today to partake in the values of equality?

All experiences are marked with invisible archetypal learning opportunities that contribute to our psyche's development and healing. Our personal healing contributes to the healing of our ancestors. The lessons are invisible to the logical mind—even though the logical mind can assimilate some reasonable rational assumptions from these experiences. Beyond our personal impressions of emotions and memories is a symbolic realm of objective principles that underlies the workings of the universe and all that evolves in this universe. The archetypal themes contain these objective principles of development and lead us past our subjective emotional reactions of vengeance and hurt.

My healing journey started with the sense that my life is a mourning process for all that went wrong in South Africa. I unconsciously held the cultural shadows in my sense of shame that resulted in excessive humility, inferiority, and alienation. I felt undeserving and guilty. In fear of stepping on anyone else's rights, I struggled to assert myself. I became a silent, confused, unacknowledged, and wounded rebel searching to belong and be whole.

How we experience—and what we perceive happens in the outside world—is often what we perceive and focus on in our nuclear family. I saw all the conflict in life. Conflict surrounded me at school and at home. My parents were intelligent and unconventional but fought constantly. I found myself either mediating or hiding from the abrasion of wounding words flying between them.

I was ten and my brother was eight when my six-year-old sister and baby brother died within six months of each other. They had separate illnesses. Death was an inconsolable crisis to my parents. Instinctively, I took responsibility to hold space for my mother's overwhelming sorrow. I withdrew further believing that it would be unfair to her to disturb her with my needs. I became invisible. Silence was my solace. My need for attachment drew me into conversations with God—who parented me.

The archetypal themes of my psychological experiences were about finding meaning. My life presented me an opportunity to understand the meaning of conflict, pain, shame, and healing. Part of the archetypal process to find meaning is the discovery of silence and tuning in. The ability to tune in teaches us to distinguish between the rules of the ego-world and the principles of the spirit. The spirit principles guide the way to healing.

Tuning In

I deeply longed for knowledge and wanted to understand the mechanisms of life. I suspected there was a world full of stimulating information just beyond the hills of isolating Mondeor. I longed to go beyond the horizons to expand my awareness. The Mondeor hills transformed to faraway places in my mind's eye. It was only a matter of time before I would actually be there. Even Bible stories and comic books stimulated my imagination. I identified with the characters of Little Lotta and Dot. Everything in my life became allegorical. Symbolism stirred and inspired my soul. My inner world stood in vast contrast to, and became more real to me, than what I encountered every day. I could sense a world beyond words. People's words sometimes move me deeply but also deceive me. Actions were rarely in agreement with people's words. I lived in an inauthentic, inconsistent and false social reality which scarred my ability to trust. Stories, on the other hand, revealed a greater world where consequences and depth of motive showed clearly. I fell silent in introversion where I contemplated the question of how to identify truth which presented many, some good and some painful, experiences in my learning.

One of my heroes, Little Lotta, ate a lot. She was a chubby girl, but she held enormous strength with which she saved those in need and solved practical problems in her environment. She was a confident and outspoken champion among her peers. I admired her and wished that I could be as spontaneous and courageous as her. My other hero was Dot. True to her name, she had a passion for dots and saw dots in everything: the stars in the sky, the stones on the ground, and the ripples on the water. Life was a big dot—a big circle where everything, all the dots, connected. All the diverse dots came together in unity to form one universe for imaginative, creative, and inventive Dot. She inspired her friends with wit and intelligence to see the magic in life. Brave, confidant Lotta and witty, brainy Dot motivated me to perceive life's virtues which filled my life with new and exciting possibilities. I strived for courage, equality, and wisdom. The Bible was equally rich with mysterious metaphors that promised significance in seemingly meaningless everyday reality. If only I could discover the meaning in the mysteries of life, I would be able to trust, and hope.

The unsettling ever-present conflict of daily life made me question the reason for the existence of dissonance. I knew that the answer could only be found on a deeper, divine, level of existence. There must be a truth, bigger than my human nature could perceive and how could I reach it? Over time, the answers became clearer as my psyche became versed in communicating with my inner world. Divine presence stared back at me in the symbolism of everyday life; I just needed to recognize it. Starry nights, storm clouds, broken twigs, windblown Transvaal grasses, the scent of ripe tomatoes in rich African soil, and the fresh squirt of juice as an orange peel cracks open, all held meaningful messages in symbols. Curious about my enlightening experiences during contemplations of readings, I longed to talk with someone about my experiences. I hoped to find a likeminded community by attending the community church. My parents focused on the practical reality of physical and financial survival, while I dwelled in the world of the spiritual in search for understanding and connection with knowledge. They slept on Sunday mornings while I walked the two or so kilometers to attend the church service. Every word read or spoken from the pulpit entranced me with reflection. The church service was pleasant enough and put me in the company of ideas, people, and beautiful organ music which to me was whispers of compassion. I considered different versions of meaning in contrast to the minister's sermon. I held internal conversations with the divine but did not express any of these ideas openly out of fear of banishment. I felt alone in the company of people but extremely rich in an unmentionable relationship with inner dimension.

Alone at home, I sometimes wrote my ideas and feelings on little pieces of paper and fed them into the air vent in the wall of my bedroom. The notes fell into the gap between the inside and outside walls of our brick house. I shared my thoughts with an invisible audience in a nowhere land between the symbolic walls of my inner and outer existence. No one in my outer hostile and inconsistent world could ever know or understand how I felt. I was an alien in that world and dared not speak to reveal my inner life.

One particular passage in the Bible always stood out with great significance to me. It influenced my entire worldview. Even if you do not understand the language, I want to share the Afrikaans version of the scripture here.

> *Want nou sien ons deur n spieël in n raaisel, maar eendag van aangesig tot aangesig. Nou ken ek ten dele, maar eendag sal ek ten volle ken, net soos ek ten volle geken is.* (1 Corinthians 13:12)

My own simple translation and personal understanding goes like this:

> Now (in this specific moment in time and space on earth), I perceive life as a riddle in a mirror, because my ego can only see one part of life at a time. However, one day, when God who knows me fully reveals life in its completeness, I will know the whole truth, fully, as it really is.

This means that God is in me and already knows all that is, but I cannot fully understand what I experience while I perceive reality only from my subjective perspective. My human ego perceives only parts of a complex reality in any specific given moment. My God-self exists at the same time as my personality. In time, I will learn to perceive this divine aspect of reality with its understanding of the whole and the full and complete truth of who I am, which my personality struggles to see. My personality needs the blind-of-spirit experience to learn from, as long as I connect it eventually to my spiritual dimension. The personality's comprehension of true reality is not complete until the personality allows the God-self within to reveal all the parts, the full picture, of our nature and our life's growth processes.

The two official English versions of this same text are as follows:

> From the Weymouth New Testament, 1 Corinthians 13:12. *The Excellence of Love: For the present we see things as if in a mirror, and are puzzled; but then we shall see them face to face. For the present the knowledge I gain is imperfect; but then I shall know fully, even as I am fully known.*

> From John Wesley's Bible Commentary Notes for 1 Corinthians 13:12. *The Excellence of Love: Now we see - Even the things that surround us. But by means of a glass—or mirror, which reflects only their imperfect forms, in a dim, faint, obscure manner; so that our thoughts about them are puzzling and intricate, and everything is a kind of riddle to us. But then—we shall see, not a faint reflection, but the objects themselves, face to face. Distinctly. Now I know in part, even when God himself reveals things to me, a great part of them is still kept under the veil. But then I shall know even as I also am known in a clear, full, comprehensive manner; in some measure like God, who penetrates the center of every object and sees at one glance through my soul and all things.*

I find these passages so thought provoking. Through the years I constantly wondered about them and concluded that our emotionally driven personality must be prejudiced to only perceive its conditioned ideas and subjective interpretations of experience. It is impossible for the personality to perceive objectively unless one bypasses one's biases. Our emotional nature conditions us to act and perceive in patterns that we repeat and therefore keep us wounded. We need to learn to perceive from a place in our psyche that is not ego-driven or affected by our history or the stories that propagate false assumptions of our experiences that keep us in these psychological wounds. We are so subjectively absorbed in our human emotions during our life experiences that it is difficult for us to see beyond our instinctive and provoked conditioned sensitivities. We can break the repeating instinctive, conditioned, emotional reactions by practicing awareness of our prejudiced assumptions by cultivating an objective view with that part of our self that is outside of our ego—our inner spiritual perspective. We access this part of our God-nature by tuning in.

It is easier to live without fear when we access the big picture of our spiritual nature. Our soul-spirit connects with all the pieces of life that serve our growth. It never intends to punish us, but we do not perceive life in such a way because our personalities believe that life is difficult. Our personalities therefore design strategies to control life in some way or other. Awareness of our specific habits and inner feelings from our spirit's perspective helps us become more objective. On the other hand our conditioned ideas tell us an emotional story that allows our instincts to react from our ego's point of view, while the core of our soul-spirit tells quite another. Our ego-interpretations of experiences are usually assumptions that confirm faulty social training; they are tainted with wounds that keep us in those wounds. Our soul-spirit has the ability to reach beneath the ego agenda for spiritual understanding and love that heals us and allows us to develop and evolve in consciousness.

The truth that we access in our spiritual faculties is more objective and it completes the logical perspective of our understanding. Only half our nature functions when we use our rational faculties only. While our personalities defensively struggle with self-interest and survival, our soul-spirits reaches toward the integration of all that exist which opens up endless possibilities of development. Our soul-spirits challenges us to interpret experiences and act with awareness that helps us develop beyond our repetitive emotional patterns. Suffering and discomfort puzzles our personality until we recognize how we lose and trap ourselves in defensive survival patterns with faulty ideas.

The relationship between our egos and our souls is a beautiful mystery that brings our ego to a place where, to its surprise, truth unfolds unexpectedly, despite its powerful attempt to control us by keeping us unconsciously trapped in our wounding ideas. Sometimes, after resisting and denying one's spiritual impetus, realities surface that are more in line with one's true essence. Without connecting to our soul-truth, our personality's identities remains mired in pride and personal ambition. We become authentic as our egos accept the identity of our soul.

The raw face of truth requires humility from our egos. Our egos must acknowledge our human as well as our divine facets as part of our nature. This humble acceptance of the noble and the corrupt potential of oneself and life is an enlightening experience for the ego. We are dark and light woven into one. Our shadows will always be part of being human but, because of them, we discover the virtuous as we tune into our divinity. We live in a dance between these two possibilities as we learn to move forward in our evolution.

In my search to understand and know more, I studied social work and psychology. The inner world of the psyche and spirituality drew me into its mystery. I devoured books which I consider as my most valuable possessions. Truth awakes in me as I contemplate the thoughts of thinkers. To avoid alienation, I had to be invisible in my society. During my youth, books were the first to give me hope by describing concepts I could relate to but could never talk about openly. I also knew that objective reality shone through, not in the exact words of any author, but in my contemplation of the essence beyond the written words. Reading contemplatively by tuning in, helped me distinguish the subjective from what is beyond the author's human abilities. Every author carries a message beyond his or her ego. Tuning in, helps us to hear that messages from our souls. Let your soul speak to you between the lines of the written word. You may discover the most amazing realizations in a book and when you read it years later you are surprised that you cannot find the same insights anywhere. This happens because your soul used the book to talk to you. You learned what you needed to at that particular time because you employed your soul and not only your reason when you read the book.

Consciousness evolves through experience as we mature on a personal and collective level. As we develop, we understand more and better and can refine our ability to listen internally. Tuning in becomes a refined instrument that detects our soul's truth. In science, the instruments used for measuring and observing theory measure what the observer's consciousness is capable of confirming at the time of measurement. The observer only measures what is already known at the moment of measurement. It is therefore important to listen beyond what you already know.

If our level of consciousness limits our ability to understand, how do we grow beyond our status quo? I believe it is vital that we listen for new and surprising information we do not expect from our souls. We have to go beyond the ego-tendency to preserve the familiar stories that echo our conditioned socialized understandings. It is also important to verify any new understandings by checking and confirming their validity. We check to verify their significance by asking our inner God-self while we observe and test these concepts in practice for their appropriateness over time.

It is important to update our perspective as we evolve and develop by letting go of old concepts and beliefs. Truth unfolds, and it will keep on changing as we grow. The unseen and complex processes the psyche undertakes are too vast to make fast assumptions about its experiences with the faculty of our personality only. Observing and testing the validity of truth is important for staying on an authentic spiritual course of healing and growth. I know many sincere seekers who deceive themselves by believing what their egos want to believe and are later disillusioned by the circumstances their faulty choices brought them. They admit that they knew in their heart of hearts the truth all along but made the wrong decisions anyway because of the temptations to settle for the needs of their egos. Exploiting our fears and desires, our egos powerfully convince us of directions contrary to our soul's interests.

Tuning in showed me that my desire to help others might seem noble, but that specific aspiration contains an element of unconscious hubris in my ego. I learned firsthand that serving others often disguises personal inner wounds while the focus is on helping others. This is an avoidance of facing one's responsibility to heal first. Our personality tricks us easily with what seems like spiritual virtues. What we want to give is what we first need to find in ourselves.

While our soul-spirit is unconscious, experiences in life challenge us and overwhelm our personalities. Then, when we tune inward to connect with our God-self, we discover unexpected insights in those unpleasant challenges. Going through a divorce was such a moment for me. This experience redirected my focus completely from living life much to the conditions that society prescribed. I was a good person, got married, and had a child, a career and worked hard to obtain material wealth. All these conventional ideals immediately broke down into a meaningless state of confusion and disillusionment when my marriage failed. I was humbled. No matter how I planned and willed my life, there was a factor beyond my doing that changed all my plans. I had to find out why. This unexpected turn of events challenged me to connect with my truth. I was living who I was not. I was living what society wanted me to be and I did not know that. At first, it was very scary to take the road indicated by my soul, but eventually I knew that the truth in my soul is my only true life. The least-expected circumstances challenged me to open my soul again. My soul steered me in a direction different from where my rational mind believed it should be.

The incomprehensible curveballs life throws at us when we least like or expect it, is in reality our unconscious mind talking to us. It is our soul desperately trying to guide us. Our crisis helps us leave our familiar psychological terrain and enter into our soul where we learn from our internal conflict. We see what we hide from ourselves. Crisis wakes us from our sleep to our inner truth, and presents us with a choice to follow our new insight. The action we need to take usually scares us beyond reason. Truth scares our egos. Truth expects us to give up security, status, possessions, and sometimes love—everything our egos tell us that we need to survive.

The challenge to go beyond our current fears and beliefs is so great that it seems impossible to accomplish. Step off the cliff of your safe ideas into the precipice of perceived danger anyway, and you will find yourself on a bridge to a new world where your sprit wants to be. Surrender to the very act you fear most. Trust your soul-spirit's truth. The unknown, where truth takes you, is a better option than the torment of emotional death when you stay in the half-truth of your conditioned and fearful personality. A miraculous and adventurous passage always appears when we act on spiritual truth. A crisis creates the precise opportunity that our souls needs for revelation and development.

There is a great struggle between our inner truth and our ego-driven personalities. Our egos works toward keeping us conditioned for the sake of our human survival and uses defensive drives in an attempt to protect us from what it was trained to perceive as threats and hurt. Our defense mechanisms start to operate the moment we become aware of emotional, physical, psychological, or social discomfort. Our egos resist the unconscious messages of our souls by preoccupying itself with survival thoughts and socially conditioned ideas that maintain past emotional patterns. Ironically, it perpetuates hurt and pain in this way. However, this very discomfort—whether it takes the form of physical symptoms, emotional pain, or conflict—speaks about important unconscious truths from our souls that demand our attention. Our well-developed egos overrule our personalities with its schemas. This is why it is important to learn how to tune inwards and listen to our soul-spirit sides. Our personalities are capable of regarding our souls' guidance when they observe the subtle information buried in the symbolism of our discomforts.

Our souls guide us to grow, heal, and evolve. Tuning in, help us discover the path towards growth. Discomfort indicates our soul's desire to move beyond our personality's desire to hold the status quo. Our egos do not easily accept new insight, ideas, or attitudes, especially when these differ from conditioned beliefs and assumptions. Nevertheless, our soul-spirit natures motivate our personalities to heal through change by unconsciously exposing us into uncomfortable circumstances and symptoms that prompt us to adjust. As long as we resist adjusting our attitudes and perceptions, we keep on making the same mistakes and history repeat itself. Our outer world resembles our ego-personalities, and our inner world resembles our divine sides.

The story of our souls is often a riddle to our personalities. Our minds and souls often contradict each other. Our minds prefer to perceive conditioned societal beliefs and our souls prefer to direct us to evolve from our current understandings. Concurrence between our souls and our personalities creates peace within us that fosters peace in the world around us. As we attend to our internal conversations with our souls, just as we listen so attentively to our personalities, we stimulate this new reality of cooperation between the parts of our nature. Conversations between our soul-spirit parts and our rational parts help these two diverse realities of logic and symbolism to work in partnership within us and open our psyches to new growth.

Clear and definite collective archetypal patterns and themes take us through spiritual developmental processes that are bigger than personal survival drives. Being aware of the symbolism that point toward these archetypal processes helps us find meaning in our everyday experiences. We make sense of painful human challenges by observing and contemplating the archetypal essences in our experiences. Painful experiences are healing opportunities. Our pain contains the riddle that informs us of the medicine we need to heal. Healing involves our full participation in life without resistance or wanting to change our experiences. In the very moment of complete acceptance of our experience, spiritual illumination unexpectedly emerges—and we hear our true voice above the arguments of our personalities. The pain we encounter in our experiences forces us to surrender to the messages of our souls when we are willing to tune into and hear the truth in our inner place of silence.

CHAPTER 3
Finding My Drop-of-God

When we tune in we find God and when we find God in us we find meaning.

Many of us often wonder about the purpose of our struggles in life. Why do we suffer? Why are we here? What is life all about? Is there any meaning in life?

Looking back on my life, I notice that everything that ever happened to me, especially the crises, contributed to a deeper understanding and to the changes that improved my reality. The path to consciousness is paved with discomfort. Personal crises are an unavoidable part of personal growth and part of our evolutionary development, but when crises or distresses make us vulnerable, we do not always know why they happen or what to do about them. How do we find our *drop-of-God* during times of crises?

At the start of our life journey, we focus on achieving the most likely goals that fulfill our central human needs. We feel utterly discouraged when obstacles obstruct the way to our dreams. Just as we think we begin to understand life, unexpected challenges confront previous understanding and require us to stretch our maturity. Many of us seek help in desolate moments. Embarrassed and fearful, we think that psychological distress is socially unacceptable and a sign of weakness. We feel it is socially expected of us to control our lives by maintaining perfect balance at all times. Societal idealism teaches us to believe that something must be wrong with us when we have problems. We feel frustrated and ashamed. We sense that we do not have a proper map or manual that guides or explains the rules and processes of overcoming hardships. Some of us notice that the guidelines that we think we have to help us manage life keep on changing anyway as we change. How do we proceed with wisdom during our upsetting, emotional turning points?

Psychological distress is nothing other than spiritual challenges toward our evolution. Our journey here on earth is about evolving our consciousness. The dual function of our nature reinforces, on the one hand, understanding of our social personality and, on the other, our spiritual side. These two aspects of our nature seem to strive towards different directions, even though we need them both to evolve. Our personality maintains security, and our soul-spirit yearns for consciousness beyond the physical. However, when these two paths become integrated and cooperate, usually toward the latter half of our lives, we find meaning and healing in the challenges that force our change, movement, and growth. Painful life experiences shape our ability to distinguish between the rational and spiritual facets of being a human—and they support our understanding of how these facets practically interrelate.

We internalize societal ideas and think of these as our own personalities. Individuation is the process of recognizing the internal soul-spirit as different from the socialized personality. Jung describes this individuation process as "a process or course of development arising out of the conflict between the two fundamental psychic facts," namely social consciousness and spiritual unconscious.

Our personalities need to belong. Our sense of belonging makes us socially conscious and we therefore desire to become what is socially acceptable or what society prescribes for us to be. Our personalities incline toward external, socially acceptable goals and achievements. In contrast to our personalities, our soul's truth is primarily unconscious to us. The soul's truth hides as a dynamic intuitive and creative drop-of God within. Carl Gustav Jung calls it the Self.

Our personalities are in an important partnership with our true soul essences; they function together in service of growth and evolution. Without my personality, I have no spiritual vehicle and, without my spiritual self, my personality only serves its goal of social survival. Who is the pilot and director of my life, and who is the copilot of this team? Is it my personality or is it my God-self?

What Is Truth and Where Do I Find It?

When something is logical it is not necessarily true. Logic does not equal truth. Truth seems comparative to the cognitive mind because it is interested in facts. The truth our souls want us to know is specifically appropriate for the growth we undergo at a specific time and place. This truth comes from the God-essence inside us and not from our logical mind. Although we reason the appropriateness of certain solutions to our problems they may not be true to what our souls need us to do. How do we find this truth? How do we get to God within us?

We have both positive and negative associations about God that taint our perspective. "God" is therefore a controversial concept. We do not talk about God lightly. History demonstrates how our belief systems provoke conflict among us concerning what we understand and know or believe about God. People have been controlled, violated, and liberated in the name of God. God even serves as justification for our subjective interpretations of our spiritual concepts and the way we conduct our everyday lives. Ideas of God influence our fears, anxieties, and hopes. Ideas of God allow us to suffer contentment or contempt. We can gain enlightenment or suffer guilt. Either way, we are extremely sensitive and emotional when it comes to God and what we believe, experience, or understand. Our emotions interfere with our objective ability to distinguish between doctrine and spirituality. Our ideas of God generally depend on our cultural experiences and circumstances but have nothing to do with the true divine essence within ourselves. We find God within this divine essence inside ourselves and not in the outer world.

The society I grew up in portrayed God as an external authority. There was some punitive divinity outside of me that demanded my obedience. God was jealous, possessive, and controlling. He was masculine and expected blind obedience and loyalty, much like the government. The political and religious leaders as well as the fathers in our community held equal authority to God. Severe punishment was a consequence for breaking any social or religious laws. This particular idea of God strongly affected the social psyche of my time. Our social consciousness of that time operated according to this particular world view.

The concept of God promoted by my society said more about the leaders and the collective state of human consciousness at the time than the true nature of whom and what God is. This patriarchal attitude of an all-powerful, self-righteous, punishing force who expected unquestioned compliance, obedience, and loyalty under the guise of protector inhibited our inner spiritual worlds. It resulted in not having any sense of freedom of thought or speech. Objective ideas were rare because of censorship and the control of information. An unspoken taboo prevented any disagreement with religious and political ideals. Authoritarianism stunts people's development and internal accountability for their choices and behavior. This world view promoted external authority and power instead of internal control and responsibility. People believe in such circumstances like these that someone external to them is in control of their lives and determines what is right and wrong for them. They also believe that God is outside of them. This misconception clearly deludes us of our very nature and robs us of our indispensable connection with our divine sides.

When leaders—government, church, or otherwise—do not allow open communication, thoughts, or opinions, people feel oppressed, submissive, or rebellious because any form of disobedience meets with overt and covert threats of rejection and exile. There is no compassionate attachment possible between people in a psychological environment that feeds the victim-oppressor dynamic through control, fear, and punishment. Authorities judged individuals with established, prejudiced ideas without considering people's opinions or outlooks. This scenario happens in societies but also in families and small groups.

Some people overdevelop a sense of guilt and responsibility because of this oppressive worldview, and others become ruthlessly self-serving. In varying degrees, this collective patriarchal attitude applied around the world during that particular century. The consequences are noticeable in the general difficulty people have with connecting in personal and cultural relationships. We do the same within our own psyche when there is no open communication between our divine side and the ego-state aspects of our personalities. As it is within individuals, it is so for groups; as it is for groups, it is so for cultures, nations and humanity.

God is the all-loving, all-inclusive essence of creative life force and consciousness in every being and aspect of creation. Every human person has God essence. God in us is the creative divine principle of life itself.

Our egos overrule our psyches with the authority and power of threat and desire. It dominates our thoughts and feelings until we hurt and long for solving our misery and blindness. Our souls silently longs for our personalities to accept God as part of us. Our personalities need to share control and cannot be the only authority over our lives. When crises exhaust our emotions, willpower, and reason, our personalities' defenses collapse enough for us to become willing and ready to perceive experience from a spiritual perspective outside of the usual viewpoints of our personality. At first, our divinity feels like a drop-of-God. As long as we know we have a drop-of-God in us, our egos move aside for us to obtain clearer access until we feel this drop become a fountain of love and light that heals, guides, and frees us from being stuck in repetitious behavior. Discovering and connecting with our God-self empowers our true nature. We find how to grow and evolve in sync with divine principles of development instead of being subservient to our fearful egos.

The Complete Collapse of My World as I Knew It

After the birth of my son, I realized that my marriage was falling apart. My baby exposed all the hidden and ignored cracks in my relationship. The birth of our child opened the wounds of our suppressed childhoods. Our wounds colored our perceptions of and reactions to each other, repeating the patterns of our parents' and cultural relationships.

Despite our training as psychologists, neither of us could communicate our true feelings. Our problems, however, were deeper than being able to communicate. The inability to communicate with our own inner selves suppressed our deep unconscious wounds. I rationalized and justified his and my behavior. My training in cognitive techniques closed me to my early experiences in childhood where I was able to access higher awareness. I forgot—and had no idea how to access—the deeper unconscious wounds and ability to heal while I focused on keeping my socially acceptable world intact. I work harder to fix things. I hoped to get approval and affection by earning recognition for my efforts. Battling intense isolation and a sense of disconnection, I tried to be a perfect wife and mother, focusing on my role instead of the origin of the unhappiness in my soul. My ego protected the fact that my partner disappointed me. We were both in denial and I made excuses for him so that I did not have to face my truth. I felt guilty for knowing that something was wrong. An internal conflict started between believing my partners' promises and believing what my soul knew. My soul desperately urged me to peek through the shroud of ego-pretense, but it suited my personality's need to stay in an idealized world because I feared the consequences of my truth. At that stage of my life, I had committed completely to my outer life and outer rewards—and ignored my inner nudging.

Truth eventually surface and cannot sustain a false relationship. The power of truth liberates. Trust your inner knowing above the invention you want to believe of what another person tells you or you tell yourself. When you commit to the truth, your judgment becomes clear. The nagging sense of discomfort that tried to warn me of something wrong turned out to be valid! I was not crazy. The nudge of discomfort started to unveil deeper and deeper layers of truth in the hidden corners of my soul and initiated me for another step in the journey toward my truth and healing. Something had to break in my ordinary life to wake my awareness of discrepancies between what I was told was true and what was real within me. The crisis was no longer about our relationship or about what or who was right or wrong but about the challenge to find my truth. I started to question every value and belief I held. I needed to find my souls true destiny.

I recognized that I had stepped into the very trap that I noticed during my childhood about society being inauthentic and had wanted to avoid so much. The shock of what I was doing made me feel like a beginner. I had entered my thirties, but I felt as if I understood and knew nothing. I was completely lost. This feeling of being a beginner often happens with spiritual awakenings or new steps in growth. My desperation evoked a humble willingness to listen and grow. This is a necessary attitude for tuning into our inner selves. I became quiet once again as I had been during childhood. My drop-of-God became audible again. I listened. My spirit started to assert over my personality. I reconnected with God in me. Owning my inner God-authority gave me the clarity and courage to step into the unknown, scary as it was for my ego.

I vowed that I would be attentive to discrepancies between the words and behavior of the people I surrounded myself with as well as the discrepancies between my soul and my personality. *I will attend to what our interaction feels like and seems like. I will attend to my deepest intuition. I will especially attend to the discrepancies within me about what I sense and what I want to believe.* The issues in my relationships are not about forgiving and understanding mistakes or bad behavior; they are about the quality of my connections and the regard we exercise for each other within those attachments. Love is not enough. Verbal apologies or even the proclamation of good intentions is not enough if it means that I allow another to neglect accountability for growing together.

When we feel something is wrong, it is. Sensing a lack of clear boundaries or a lack of clear overt commitment from a partner might be the issue that causes discomfort in your attachment. That does not necessarily mean that our worst fears are real, but it does mean that we have detected subtle internal conflicts that need resolve and clarification. Listen to those internal soul nudges. Emotions take up so much space in our lives that we cannot hear our spiritual truths. Silence the voices of emotion and convention and listen to hear your drop-of-God.

I knew that I had to stop giving people outside of me authority to control my happiness. This adjustment helped my personality not to feel bruised by what I perceived as deception. I discovered and acknowledged my inner power and value. Experiences of deception were necessary challenges for me to make this adjustment. There are unexpected gifts in every painful life experience. False love paradoxically reveals true love; deception reveals truth, and conflict, peace. Every action I took in the direction of my souls guidance strengthened my courage and trust in life because the results confirmed an authentic inner truth—no more discrepancies or conflict.

CHAPTER 4

Once More into the Abyss

T en years after I left my first marriage I confronted an unexpected challenge with my new family. Life had finally settled or so I thought. My soul had other plans for me.

Warnings of approaching danger startled me at night through haunting dreams. I ignored these attempts of my inner voice to reach me. My soul spoke louder through circumstances by exposing me to actual encroaching violent events. Escaping physical danger with hair-raising closeness a couple of times, I started to listen to my soul's calling, but I did not like what I heard. I was prompted by my dreams and visions to leave my country. I resisted and denied this message by rationalizing and denying it to myself as hard as I could. I faced an even more fundamental challenge than leaving my marriage. Now I faced having to leave my country. I realized that each crisis in my life prepares me to move even further beyond my boundaries if I am willing to take a leap of faith by trusting my inner guidance. My new husband trusted my inner guidance and stood committedly united with me in our spiritual journey. My journey is his and his, mine.

The Beckoning

Sometimes an image in front of us beckons to wake us up to new spiritual frontiers, but our slumber of assumed comfort keeps us unconscious and unable to recognize it. How do we recognize and respond to these subtle messages of our souls? How do we distinguish, trust, and act with confidence on this guidance?

A dream, a person, or an experience might hold the key to confirming the messages from our higher selves. The messages of our souls want to connect with our rational will and understanding—and then lead us to the next step in our life's journey if we are willing. Our souls are in tune with the need for growth and expose us to challenging experiences that break us out of our status quo. We rarely feel ready for life-altering challenges, but we have to identify them as healing opportunities to be able to use them.

My beckoning began with dreams and visions while circumstances confirmed the messages. Circumstantial confirmation shifted my attitude and my willingness to act. My mind could not anticipate the details of the miraculous unfolding of reality as doors started to open in the direction my soul needed to move. The beckoning of my soul-spirit usually begins with events that challenge me to trust an internal truth above the voices of my socialized and fearful personality. I have to be able to distinguish between what is the voice of my spirit and what of my fears and desires.

We conquer our fear and establish trust that gives us courage to act on what we know is true in our souls when we shift our perspective from what our personalities say to what our spirit urges. Trust and courage defies human logic and personal effort. From our souls perspective we need to be ready to act in an opposite direction to what our socialized personalities anticipated for us. The timing of this action depends on a convergence of circumstances. We prepare for new behavior and action by studiously observing the factors that our souls indicate through signs and symbols in our everyday life.

A Haunting Dream

The mid-nineties were a magical time in South Africa. Nelson Mandela's release from prison filled everyone with hope and joy for a new future. Mandela became president during South Africa's first true democratic election. Tired of social conflict, I welcomed the thought of being part of the new South Africa. Then I had a dream that cautioned an opposite scenario to my hopes.

In my dream, I stared out into the night, skimming my eyes over what seemed to be a body of calm water in front of me. As my eyes got used to the darkness, I saw the outline of a woman's body lying halfway in the water covered by a sheet. I came closer to make sure that what I saw was actually so. Anxiously, I pulled the sheet away to investigate her mortality. It became clear that she was dead. Then I noticed the baby next to her, struggling to breathe. There was no time to waste; I had to save the baby! I jumped in and pulled the baby from the water, urgently resuscitating it. Finally, the baby coughed and started to breathe.

I felt happy and relieved to have saved the baby and noticed for the first time what a beautiful baby it was. Without warning, the smiling baby turned into a vicious, glaring, sharp-toothed monster. Its nails became claws that dug into my body as it bit chunks of flesh from my neck with sharp, pointed teeth. I woke in a sweaty panic, shocked and confused.

The dream was vivid and disturbing. This dream was without any doubt important. I had no idea what it meant. I struggled to understand the symbolism for a long time because the usual rational psychodynamic interpretations did not feel right. For months, I tried to analyze it, this way and that, thinking that perhaps parts of my psyche was self-destructive while other parts were dying or transforming. The dream nagged me for clarity. I sought counsel from my colleagues. Their interpretations left me more confused and incomplete. Something was missing. What made sense to my mind did not make sense to my inner truth. Exhausted by the emotional turmoil, I resigned from forcing an answer to this riddle from my rational mind. I asked my God-self for answers, and my mind became quiet.

Asking questions and waiting with a silent mind for a response always works. A week or so later, I abruptly woke up one night from a deep sleep. A clear and powerful "ah-ha" struck me like lightning. Instantly clear, the dead woman in the water was my mother country. She had died. The baby was the fragile baby-state of the newborn South Africa. I supported its life, but became its victim. I was in danger and had the sense that I had to leave even though I resisted this knowledge with all my reason! This realization to leave did not come from my logical mind but was a knowing that came from my soul.

The dream revealed itself and my soul-spirit felt clear about the message, but my mind still resisted. There was no rational way to accept the threat that the new South Africa would hurt me in any way. The very thought saddened me deeply. I insisted on playing a part in breathing life into my new South Africa. There was a chance for change, and all my painful childhood memories of playground conflicts and social prejudice between various cultural groups could end in harmony. All my life, I had dreamed that people of different colors, cultures, and religions would eventually live in peace and respect. *Is this not what the new South Africa stands for? Is this not what is supposed to happen now?*

The update to the Constitution of the Republic of South Africa occurred on May 8, 1996. After two amendments, the finalized Constitution was signed into law on December 10, 1996. The process of constructing a new Constitution involved the largest public participation program ever carried out in South Africa. The final document had to be true and represented the collective wisdom agreed upon by all the South African people. It is as follows:

> We, the people of South Africa, recognize the injustices of our past; honor those who suffered for justice and freedom in our land; respect those who have worked to build and develop our country; and believe that South Africa belongs to all who live in it, united in our diversity. We therefore, through our freely elected representatives, adopt this Constitution as the supreme law of the Republic so as to heal the divisions of the past and establish a society based on democratic values, social justice and fundamental human rights; lay the foundations for a democratic and open society in which government is based on the will of the people and every citizen is equally protected by law; improve the quality of life of all citizens and free the potential of each person; and build a united and democratic South Africa able to take its rightful place as a sovereign state in the family of nations. May God protect our people. *Nkosi Sikeleli Afrika. Morena boloka setjhaba sa heso. God seën Suid-Afrika.* God bless South Africa. *Mudzimu fhatutshedza Afurika. Hosi katekisa Afrika.* (The official website of the South African Government Information: http://www.info. gov.za/documents/constitution/ holds the complete Constitution document of October 11, 1996)

The allure of our county's new constitution enchanted me, and I focused on the intention of the new Constitution as the only possible reality. I hoped that our people in South Africa had reached an understanding of human cooperation and reverence. Nelsen Mandela as well as many others worked and suffered for this vision to become a reality. How could my dream tell me otherwise? I preferred to imagine that the ideal in my mind was a reality, just as I had done with my first marriage. However, others and my intentions and the words of a constitution were not enough to make a vision real. Our human nature easily reverts to precious conditioned beliefs that feed our wounds and hurtful behavior. Change is not easy.

Explosive surges of violent crime began to erupt in different parts of the country. Crime was always present in South Africa to one degree or other because of deprivation and poverty, but it continued to escalate instead of dissipate. I kept on hoping that the warnings in my dream was not true and consoled myself that circumstances will soon change for the better.

However, crime did not stop but only became worse. Torture, muggings, rape, murder, and hijackings became everyday phenomena. Social problems among jobless youth must surely explain the gangs armed with their AK-47 weapons. Pockets of violent criminal groups spread fear and terror everywhere in everyone. Entitlement, racial hatred, ruthless rebelliousness, lack of education, and extreme discrepancy between the rich and poor reigned. A lack of supportive social structures ran deep in the collective psyche. Crime surges seemed to indicate a collective "shadow" of competitive tribalism and revenge.

The Shadow is a Jungian concept of denied and rejected aspects of our nature. Tribalism frequently refers to the possession of a strong cultural or ethnic identity that separates the members of one group from the members of another. It is a precondition for members of a tribe to possess a strong feeling of identity that excludes others. Just as on the playground years ago in my youth, different groups of people continued their wars. The reconciliation process did not stop the sweeping of hurts and injustices between cultures under the carpet. Everyday relationships revealed that there was still no deep-rooted resolve or healing. Not everyone was ready to embrace the principles of a new Constitution for our new South Africa. These new ideas did not bring new feelings in people. Old ideas and wounds were still unresolved. My mother country was dead as my first marriage. I was in danger and had to listen to my inner voice to become separated and independent as my dream indicated.

Dreams can be meaningful on many levels, and the same dream can reveal more truths over time as we mature our relationship with our soul-spirit essence. The dream of the dead mother and new baby relates to an archetypal symbol found in descriptions of Gerhard Dorn, a sixteenth-century alchemist. Marie-Louise van Franz analyzed his work in her book, *Alchemical Active Imagination* (Shambhala, Boston and London, 1997).

Van Franz relays Dorn's description of one of the alchemical processes we all need to experience in our development as the death of one's mother, which he calls the dragon-body of the psyche. Our dragon-body, our physical and ego self, disintegrates so that one can give birth to our divine child side, symbolic of our conscious divine-self. This divine child part of us grows and integrates with all aspects of our psyche as we transform to be a whole, in other words, a healed being. Letting go of our beliefs in the existence of life as finite and ego-centric is a necessary archetypal death that transforms us to adapt to new phases of our development. Transformation means renewal and new physical circumstances.

Significant Signs Symptoms and Synchronicities

My dream indicated a path I did not expect while my own need was about participating in helping South Africa heal. The conflict my dreams nudged me with provoked debilitating migraine headaches. My body joined in sending me signs to communicate the urgency of my soul's messages through painful symptoms I could not ignore. Searching for relief of the extreme pain, I started a simple meditation practice. All I really needed to do was listen to my inner voice but sometimes we need to go through a process of confirming our inner truth before we feel ready to act. The meditation practice was part of that confirmation process, exposing me to silence and contemplation. This time my God-self upped the ante with seriously impactful signs. During one of these ten-minute sessions, a very clear threefold vision occurred. A great Buddha appeared in the inner space between my eyes. Its extraordinarily divine presence was neither masculine nor feminine. It carried a five-pointed crown like a king. On each of the five points on the crown was an image of the same Buddha. The Buddha exerted a presence of love, peace, and wisdom. I just observed with awe, not having a clue about its meaning.

Seemingly unrelated, a second and third vision appeared rapidly. The second vision showed an ancient Egyptian man shining with intelligence. The third vision showed a group of North American Indian women dancing in a circle around a ceremonial fire. I was unfamiliar with Buddhism, Egyptians, or First Nations people. Nevertheless, the Buddha, Indian women, and Egyptian man's presences felt strangely familiar—despite the fact I had never seen anyone like this. It felt as if I knew them perfectly on a deep unconscious level. I wrote the sequence of my visions in my notebook and forgot about it.

Experience with visions, dreams, and other subtle observations have taught me that it is possible to have access to collective information. Carl Gustav Jung was clearly aware of this from his work on the collective unconscious. Jung claimed that what we categorize as mystical experiences are significant guideposts of developmental processes that can happen throughout life. These experiences connect us to the collective unconscious where we access universal truths.

When I got an invitation to attend a "Cross-Cultural Conflict Resolution" event, I welcomed the opportunity for discussion with other South Africans about the state of affairs between our peoples. Still battling the disturbing dream that jolted me to leave South Africa, I hoped and anticipated that my participation in conversations with other groups with the objective to heal our broken intercultural relationships will turn out to be so positive that my dream was just an inner fear. However, I happened to be the only white person among hundreds of black people at that event.

I was alone, representing the entire white population of South Africa and its shame-filled, wounded history. I represented not only the Afrikaner oppressor—but also all the other white groups that lived on that continent; the British, the Jewish, the Scottish and so on who did not think of themselves as racists. I participated enthusiastically in the emotionally taxing workshop. The wounds of an entire country's pain opened in me that day, connecting me to everyone who suffered on South African soil— white and black, the same. History lived in my bones like dust on the warm landscape. Stories and memories shared, triggered all forms of injustice that tore at and devoured my psyche like the destructive monster-child in my dream. At once, I was in pain with everyone present and not present.

We all carry a collective history inside as a part of our personal healing journey. Our personal circumstances symbolize relevant themes about where and in what direction our conscious attitude and behavior need to expand. I willingly involved myself in a personal as well as a collective healing process. I wanted to participate in creation by my personal healing and work for collective evolution. We are all victims as well as perpetrators of our circumstances. Sometimes we are only willing to see and identify with one of the sides. We see ourselves as victims and blame, or as perpetrators and suffer guilt. Victims and perpetrators are angry and resentful. We hardly ever recognize that we are like our enemy within ourselves. This void in our awareness keeps us at war with one another and within ourselves. History is a heavy burden of wounds we drag with us into the future and pass on to our children when we don't adjust our attitudes. Our holding onto victimhood or guilt prevents our next generations from healing too. We are too keen to open old wounds and emerge our emotions in negative thoughts by perpetuating our stories of pain on each other. Even though we should share and have compassion with each other's experiences, we are again too ready to blame and avoid accountability to contribute to the changes we need to establish together. Filled with unconscious shame or resentment, we diminish our involvement and avoid looking one another in the face.

The people present that day at the Cross Cultural Conflict Resolution workshop, faced me with a clear instruction to leave South Africa. They explained that I did not belong because I was there alone; that despite my being there that day still made it impossible for them to see and hear me. It is my white skin and my Afrikaans language that reminded them of the oppressors that were not there to participate in healing our deep cultural wounds. I was numb with apprehension and pain.

I contemplated what happened at the workshop in depth, trying to come to terms with my reality. B. Hamber talked about "The Psychological Implications of the Truth and Reconciliation Commission with Special Reference to the South African Police Services" at the Police Training College in Pretoria on May 13–15, 1996, at a conference hosted by the Center for the Study of Violence and Reconciliation that felt appropriate to me that day at the Cross Cultural Conflict Resolution workshop.

> Survivors of traumatic events, and more broadly governments in transformation from past political conflict like South Africa, are often urged to let sleeping dogs lie or to let bygones be bygones. However, psychologically sleeping dogs do not lie; past traumas do not simply pass or disappear with the passage of time. Psychologically, we cannot ignore the history and past traumas. Historic traumas will always leave emotional consequences for individuals and groups. Repressed pain and trauma generally block emotional life, have psychologically adverse consequences and can even lead to physical symptoms. Psychological restoration and healing can only occur through providing the space for survivors to feel heard and for every detail of the traumatic event to be re-experienced in a safe environment.

The workshop was an opportunity to meet and heal, but it never materialized. Healing was not yet possible because not enough people had participated in discussions that day. I was out of place to do the work as the single white representative. It was painful to accept my helplessness in this regard and let go of my sense of responsibility. I surrendered my personal agenda, idealized views of my purpose, and accepted responsibility to heal myself first. Healing me required that I act according to my inner guidance. I had to leave South Africa despite my resistance to do so.

The second I accepted the truth of my inner guidance, an effortless flow of circumstances opened all the doors to our new and unexpected destination for my family and me. There was no struggle to make anything happen. The ease in which everything unfolded confirmed that I was on the right track. Whether it be people, places, ideas, or belief, be willing to leave everything behind that does not support and serve the truth of your soul—even if your personality longs for the comfort of the familiar. When a plan comes from the soul, doors open and bridges appear where you did not expect them to be.

The Bridge Appears

I surrendered to the messages in my dreams three months after my visions of the Buddha, the Egyptian man, and the Indian women. I had no idea where to go or what to do. Canada became an unexpected option, and I set off on a journey to investigate. This trip was not about what I wanted but where my soul wanted me to be. I felt so completely disillusioned by my rational plans and ideas about life that I could only listen to my soul. Watchfully, I listened to my inner guidance every step of the trip.

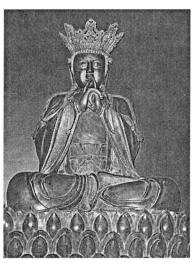

Vairocana Buddha (means light all over) Royal Ontario Museum Toronto

Canada has a gentle spirit. Most important on my list of activities was to confirm the possibility of continuing my profession with the registration bodies in Canada. Then I visited the Royal Ontario Museum. There, right in front of my very eyes, stood the Buddha of my vision! How was that possible? The first part of my vision, months earlier, manifested in front of my eyes.

Three months after my first visit, we landed in Canada as immigrants to settle in a home in Kanata, Ontario. Everyone was surprised by how fast and smooth our immigration process proceeded. We had no friends, family, or jobs in Canada. Trust in inner guidance spurred our courage and confirmed itself trustworthy.

Nine months after our arrival, I met an Aboriginal elder at the Tulip Festival in Ottawa. She invited me to a woman's gathering. The theme of the gathering was about bringing medicine back to women. Hundreds of Aboriginal women, and a few others, pitched their tents on Victoria Island in the Ottawa River. I learned that, for thousands of years, the Algonquin First Nation people had used this tiny island in the river under the shadow of Parliament Hill as a meeting place for gatherings, trading, and spiritual celebrations.

We laughed, cried, and shared our medicine through stories, gifts, and wisdom during the day. We ate, sang, and worked together with a vibrant sense of solidarity. We attended a sweat lodge. At night, we joined in fire and pipe ceremonies, and we slept in tents under a starry sky. We accepted and appreciated one another's differences through sharing our diverse experience as a medicine we developed in our souls. I realized that another part of my vision of months before was unfolding in front of my eyes.

Each woman brought something to burn at the fire ceremony, to release the past. Some silent and others prayed audibly asking the Divine Source for support and guidance in healing of self as well as the whole community and all people of the earth. The Divine Source was whomever that might be for you—God, Jesus, the Creator, the Blessed Virgin, the Great Mother, spirit, the universe, the archangels, the saints, or guardian angels. As the energy from the past was released symbolically in the smoke by the burning of material or symbolic articles, we silently supported each other in healing, replacing the wounds with love and acceptance. For the first time in my life, I felt nurtured by a community. I knew I had found my place of belonging. I had found "home."

In the North American Indian tradition, an eight-pointed star is a sacred symbol that often appears on handcrafted quilt blankets. The elder, Kayendres, made such a quilt as a special gift for one woman to take home at the end of the weekend. Everyone wanted this handmade quilt with the significant Aboriginal eight-pointed star. To my surprise, she drew my name from the bag of names. I approached the stage to receive this special blanket during the closing ceremony. No one knew me.

Kayendres wrapped the blanket around my shoulders like a sacred garment and smudged me with an eagle feather. Smudging is a purification ceremony, which involves the burning of sacred herbs—sage, sweet grass, and cedar—in a special shell bowl. Smoke from the herbs is distributed over the body of the recipient of the smudging, with a feather by the elder, purifying the thoughts, eyes, ears, and voice so that one will only think, see, hear and speak truth. A sense of incredible love, grace, and honor humbled me. My ideal of a lifetime became a reality in that moment. Robbed of their homes and language in their own country, the Aboriginal people of Canada welcomed me "home" with a sacred blanket symbolizing peace and cooperation. I honor my spiritual family. They are the carriers of true spiritual healing.

This star-blanket was especially significant to me because of its symbolic meaning. It illustrated a vision that represented the four colors (black, red, white and yellow) of the peoples in the world uniting as a whole. The symbol carries hope for this spiritual ideal of peaceful integration of different aspects of humanity. This integration and cooperation also applies to couples, families, and communities.

Although the Archetypal theme many of us deal with are the same, each of us find uniquely individual answers true to us personally that activate our behavior choices.

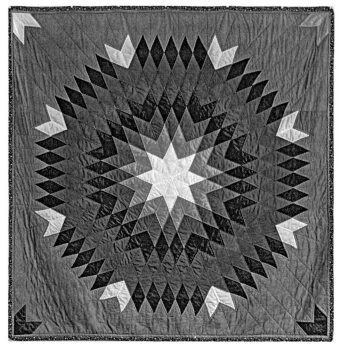

The eight-pointed star-blanket, sacred North-American Indian symbol

Receiving this blanket was a spiritual homecoming ceremony. Inspired by the moment after the smudging, I spontaneously invited the only black and yellow sister present in the group to join Kayendres and me. I threw the blanket over us all to symbolize unity. The entire gathering of woman responded with cries of joy for the visual confirmation of the four cardinal principles in the Native tradition which I did not know about consciously at that moment: respect for Wakan Tanka (the sacred or the divine, the Great Spirit), respect for Mother Earth, respect for our fellow men and women, and respect for individuals. I have found my new motherland of healing. Kayendres named me "Woman Who Sees in the Dark."

Act on true inner guidance and the bridge appears. Every day is an adventure in expanding awareness and healing.

CHAPTER 5

Healing Principles

T hroughout various developmental stages of our life, we experience discomfort and conflict in a variety of forms. Physical symptoms, circumstances, emotions, and relationship problems are expressions of psychological discomfort represented to our minds by our unconscious. Puzzled by these symptoms, we are indeed challenged to heal by attaining the truth that underlies the symbolism in these symptoms.

Our practical life serves as a mirror that holds up a deeper truth of our nature when we are ready to recognize it. The divine in us lies in the objective collective of our unconscious. From here, our spirit attempts to communicate to our conscious mind through the physical expressions of our psyche. Understanding and accepting the purpose and function of the unconscious and learning how to recognize, validate, and value these messages from our soul is necessary for our healing.

The Principles

Expect Feedback and Signs

Everything in life is feedback. Our responses to all the stimuli we encounter in our life experiences are the feedback we need to contemplate understanding. What we perceive in our outside world mirrors images of our psyche. This feedback is not necessarily verbal, expressed, or received rationally. Our psyches register responses to every experience we encounter. These responses can be psychosomatic or sensational. Our unconscious triggers unexpected behavior coincidences or dreams that are also significant.

Acknowledgment that the presenting issues are meaningful allows the unconscious to continue its push for awareness. The more we attune to the underlying meaning of events and our responses to life, the more conscious we become. Awareness of our true motives and feelings are necessary, thus we need feedback to reflect on our truth. Ordinary, everyday circumstance as well as encounters with others can lead to awareness of our soul's messages.

It was a cold day. Fall had just begun. I felt depleted and stripped of joy after a visit to my ill parents. My heart felt cold and gloomy like the empty house that I had come back to. I tried to heat the house by notching up the thermostat on the heating system. No increase of heat was noticeable. I checked. The pilot light was out. There was no one to ask for help. My husband, friends, and neighbors were all away on travels. What could I do?

An urgency to get warm forced me to find information about the functions and workings of a pilot light. Researching methods to light the pilot in my furnace suddenly struck a chord. My spirit-light was out! The flame of internal support—my connection to trust and inspiration that kept life meaningful and warm—had died down. I had allowed sad past memories to rob me of my light; my God-self. The past can do that.

Sometimes I visit and stay for a while in the dark cold winds of the past—with the traumatic complexities and wounds it contains. It pulls me down with its heavy hands until I sink into a dark pit of unkind aching that does not want to release its clutches. When allowing myself to indulge in old emotions, my light blows out. As long as the light of objectivity burns and can ignite fast after the moment it goes out, my inner home—my psyche—should never get cold and dark. When my personality loses perspective, that fire does not want to burn. This mundane experience gave me awareness upon reflection. I realized that putting my attention on the past, more than necessary for growth to emerge, pulls me empty of life force. I realized that the past is only helpful to me as long as it serves as building blocks for understanding to help me heal and grow. Heal and Glow.

Practice Awareness by Contemplating Observations

Notice the signs and symbolism in synchronicities and symbolic events like dreams, and then contemplate them by waiting while asking questions about how they apply to our current learning. They are signposts that lead us to the truth where we find new meaning and direction for growth.

Healing requires the practice of honest, patient self-awareness. We need silence to contemplate our honest hidden responses to experiences. Our egos construct defenses to prevent us from seeing the hard psychological truth, and we need to practice the ability to accept the truth underneath our defensiveness. The symbolic riddles that underlie the scenes of our everyday life reveal this truth.

Contemplation of the symbolism promotes the resolution of the riddles in our experiences. The truth is sometimes unexpected or shocking in its surprising revelations. The truth awakens us from the contentment of the lies our conditioning has taught us to believe and repeat to ourselves. However, never make fast conclusions. Allow the truth to unfold and confirm it as you stay attentive to the signs.

A woman dreamed that her ex-husband was very angry with her. A couple of days later, she observed two men fighting over a son in the street. One of the men was the boy's biological father, and the other was the stepfather. Frustrated about how each of them was preventing the other from having a relationship with the boy, they violently blamed and accused each other with forceful punches.

The woman noticed her emotional response of concern and sadness for the men—and especially the child—and immediately asked her God-self how this related to her. During meditation, she recognized the similarity of the street scene and her reality. She realized how her ex-husband might have resentment toward her and her current husband about their son. She immediately communicated her gratitude toward her ex-husband, recognizing his love for their son and his generosity of spirit to share his son with another man. She also reassured him that, while their son appreciates his stepfather, he also appreciates and will always love his biological father. Nothing can change that.

Recognition of others and their emotional turmoil is important. Giving love and acceptance to everyone in your life—even if you do not agree with their behavior—is just as important because our children suffer our conflicts if we do not repair them. This woman showed regard for the subtle messages of what her soul-spirit was trying to tell her through her dream and the synchronistic event that stirred her emotions.

Accept What Is

Whatever "is" is necessary for wisdom to mature. A powerful paradox is present in the process of acceptance. When we accept what we most despise and resist, we find that we heal. Most of us think, or at least hope, that when we get rid of what we do not want, we will change in ways that will take away all our problems. Even though it seems logical, getting rid of what we do not like is not the answer for healing. The qualities our ego does not like will continue to be part of the composition of our human nature.

Have you ever tried to get rid of a trait you do not like in yourself? We cannot get rid of any part of ourselves. The more you try—by suppression, repression, or forced effort—the more the trait persists. It even becomes exaggerated. Our souls know this and do not agree with our minds in this regard. The strange thing is that our souls are right! Once accepted, the trait softens. What we completely accept without fighting against heals. The reason for this is that the part we do not like operates like a hurt child within our personalities. This part needs love and acceptance from our God-self, the center of our psyche, to relax its efforts to get our attention with its negative feelings and behavior. Wounded feelings heal when we embrace them instead of rejecting or criticizing ourselves for feeling what we do.

For example, when we have a tendency to feel easily hurt, we tend to withdraw. By learning to accept the hurting side of us with understanding, that part does not have to react so forcefully. Any withdrawing part is a desire to protect the ego from perceived hurt. Knowing how this part came about by considering how your history promoted its coming into existence can help you choose to live with compassion for your human nature without defensive reactions.

You can practice exercising courage to act opposite to the withdrawing defense by moving toward others instead of away. The new behavior helps the wounded aspect heal. Healing helps. We connect with others instead of perpetuating the wounding idea and response. As it becomes easier to engage instead of withdraw, we understand that the hurt part of ourselves responded to its conditioned pattern, which kept it in an emotional hurt cycle. This new perspective and new experience turn our ways around. The tendency to withdraw might creep up on us occasionally, especially when we feel vulnerable, but our willingness to practice and develop new behavior heals our unconscious repetitive patterns. We feel free and liberated.

Another example is our ability to retaliate angrily when we feel defensive in relationships. This is another way of defending against unconscious vulnerability. Anger and aggression toward others is a projection of a fear of being vulnerable. In this case, we may have to learn to acknowledge our internal frustration before we project it onto another. Loving our vulnerable side allows us to choose a calm, objective, conscious standpoint—instead of acting out with aggression—toward people around us.

Think of it this way. Instead of taking away what you consider to be bad, why not add to your life what nurtures and nourishes you? Instead of trying to eat as little as possible when you want to lose weight, add more vegetables, fruits, and nuts that nourish you. Instead of getting rid of parts of yourself, give yourself understanding and love. Love, acceptance, and nourishment allow you to blossom.

Everything in our circumstances is exactly what we need in order to become aware of what attitude to change in ourselves for healing and growth. We may want to change circumstances because we feel unhappy with them, but we actually need these to teach us. Before we have learned to hear our soul's teaching that hides in those very circumstances we do not accept, there is no point in trying to change them.

Accept that everything is how it should be—and things do change only as we learn what we need to learn from those specific circumstances. Even if we willfully change circumstances, the same patterns have a tendency to reoccur if we don't use the message in the circumstances to transform our attitudes. Our inner change sets us up for external change fitting to our state of consciousness.

Distinguish between Human Ego and Divine Self

Who is talking—one of my ego-states or my God-self? Am I listening to my fear, need, desire, or truth? We are human and learn from doing human things, but we have to know that we are not only human. We have a God side that supports our human side by expressing divine principles into our humanness.

For our human life to express the divine, we need to identify what part of us is driving our behavior choices. We accept our fallibilities by identifying them as our human aspects. Then we access our God-self by choice with an awareness of how our egos manipulate our behavior. As long as we deny our humanness, our God-self cannot express itself through our physical nature because human nature on its own deems us unaware and unconscious of our divinity. Our behaviors become automatic, repetitive instincts saturated in fear patterns and misconception. The conscious distinction between our human nature and our God-self keeps us humble and aware of our imperfections but also help us be liberated from our ego's hold. Accessing our divine self, we access compassion insight and choice over behavior. Choice gives us the freedom to heal and grow.

Social learning conditions us to accept only the most ambitious and idealistic human qualities, emotions, and behavior. We deny our humanness as well as our God-self by identifying with idealistic, socially acceptable traits we believe our egos achieve. We want to be who we think we should be and lose touch with our divinity. Accept the complete package that you are. Our egos are capable of all things human and unite with our God-self to access our divine potential in order to evolve.

Ignoring and suppressing the imperfections of our human nature allows these imperfect qualities to become destructive parts Jung called *shadows*. We fear these shadows and deny that they exist within us, which gives them more unconscious power to operate in our personality. Our personality wants to rid itself of these shadow parts, while our divine core, the aware self, accepts the shadow parts as part of life that leads our awareness to find insight and healing. We cannot get rid of any part of our nature—only destructive beliefs, ideas, and behavior we choose to change because of our insight.

Fear is a powerful emotion that acts like a dictatorship in our psyches. Fear can be a shadow when it is unconscious. Fear increases our biological survival instincts by triggering flight-and-fight impulses meant to defend against perceived threats to survival. Our egos have different ideas about what those threats are, depending on what socialized ideas we identified with. Modern-day reality rarely requires life-threatening defenses, but our personality learns to detect any emotional threat to our adopted identities and activates defense mechanisms.

So instilled are the fear patterns in our social conditioning that we find it difficult to operate without perceiving these threats and reacting to them. In fact, we tune our perceptions very finely to detect threats that relate to wounding themes we encountered in our childhood, which confirm our egos identities. Conditioning also sensitizes us to be sensitive to unconscious ancestral wounds.

The defense mechanisms our personalities use regulate our reactions and actions. Consciousness of how our fears trigger our defenses helps heal our shadow parts when we choose not to act in these reactive defensive ways. A new objective perspective of differentiating between what are reactive emotions and chosen healthy behaviors, creates a nurturing and accepting attitude toward our wounds—without indulging and maintaining these. The love and acceptance we tap from our God-selves nurtures and attend to our wounds with acknowledgment for the nature of our human egos, while we allow ourselves to grow beyond these old conditioned patterns.

Our conditioned beliefs and ideas impose limitations on our abilities and potential to evolve in the same way fears do. These limitations prevent growth and healing. Lovingly pruning these limiting ideas allows us to understand how they became part of our learned behavior. We do not need to hold our growth in jeopardy.

Practice Love and Unconditional Acceptance

Unconditional love and acceptance is not a natural human ability. We tend to love what we like. Love is acceptance of all that is possible not only what we prefer. We do, however, access unconditional love through the universal divine. The God-selves inside all of us reaches out to all the negative human potential in us with unconditional acceptance.

When we act on the principle of unconditional love to heal our relationship with life, it is possible to finally truly love and accept others and ourselves. Unconditional acceptance is the ultimate father-mother, divine parent archetype, which sustains, protects, nurtures, and guides our personalities. We access this love from our inner God-selves in the objective collective unconscious. It is from here that we connect to the bigger cycles and meaning of the objective archetypal principles. It is from here that we bring the divine insight and awareness to our lives and are able to liberate ourselves from the shackles of conditioned behavior patterns that keep us in pain.

Prune and Weed Out Old Conditioned Ideas

Prune and weed out redundant beliefs and behavior—but not aspects of your nature. Weeding old ideas makes space for healthy growth. We demonstrate the principle of unconditional love internally, interpersonally, and socially through conscious choices in our actions once we connect with it. Healing and growth happens when we acknowledge and accept others and ourselves.

One's behavior may be unacceptable, but one's person always deserves acknowledgment and respect. We suffer the consequences of our own destructive behavior in order to learn to love our nature and prune our ideas and behaviors.

Understand the Bigger Scheme

There is a bigger scheme beyond our egos agendas. The rhythms of the divine universal scheme in our soul-spirits always maintain an authority over the measures of our egocentric personalities. Our egos tells us a story that impresses us with the desire for power, the ability to fix, help, possess, and know—all because of our personal effort. Our egos take on a hero role that makes us feel responsible for what happens in life.

We are indeed responsible for what we do, but only truly when we consciously participate in the unfolding evolution of our development with constructive choices. Our instinctive and defensive responses come from our egos perspective alone. Ego perspective is without awareness of the bigger scheme of the divine universe that unfolds its evolutional process regardless of our egos. It is up to us to connect with our divine aspects and cultivate awareness that incorporates cooperation between our egos and our God-selves within. We easily feel obligated or guilty when we feel incapable of managing life. Our egos have a hero complex that wants to overcome life on its own. It loses perspective because the ego believes it is operating on its own. Don't push and don't force; allow life to unfold its own patterns. Cooperate by working with the universal flow as you stay alert and willing to act on true guidance.

Collective themes from our ancestral and universal human history are part of this bigger scheme that we belong to—and they intricately weave themselves into our personal lives. We all partake in the development of consciousness collectively as we develop personally and individually. The divine archetypes are indicators of this bigger scheme that functions as the building blocks of all life in the universe that we are part of.

Heal through Partnership

We live during a time that forms history; the stories of timelines that contains and echoes collective themes. These themes resonate with the stories we also carry within us in the form of personal wounds. We recognize these themes in the types of challenges we are confronted with and need to heal. We become conscious of the qualities of the archetypal themes as personal developmental opportunities. Our community and the culture we grow up in represents us therefore with a partnership in healing through exposing us with the exact challenges for our development. We are therefore in partnership with the time and place of our life, the nation, culture, family, friends, and personal partners in order to heal. These partners stimulate awareness in all our healing processes throughout our lives.

We always find ourselves in relationships that help us understand more about life and ourselves. All relationships are partnerships where we learn about the parts of our being alive. We first encounter life's primary archetypal principles of masculine and feminine. The masculine and feminine principles and qualities are not about men and women or sexuality—but about the abstract universal qualities of action and willpower contrasting with the qualities of acceptance and nurturing. These symbolic complementary counterparts represent wholeness. Our primary guardians which are usually our parents unconsciously impress the nature of masculine and feminine principles profoundly on our psyches. This function can also befall others.

We need to know and understand the functions of both masculine and feminine qualities, of which both are present in men and women simultaneously but differently. The archetypal relationship between the masculine and feminine principles within us is the foundation of an operational spiritual truth on which we become whole and healed. It is the foundation of our ability to act and know versus our ability to accept and be silent. It is the foundation of the way we integrate the functions of our divine and logical psyche. This dynamic affects the evolution of family and every next generation's ability to grow and relate.

We are in spiritual partnership with all the people who enter our lives—siblings, friends, or enemies. Our encounters with others trigger emotional experiences that demonstrate our various ego-states. Our intimate partners are the other important personal assistants in our growth—as we are to them. We usually need acceptance, love, support, intellectual development, and happiness in these partnerships and do not think of our enemies and the people we do not like as partners. However, our enemies are especially important partners in healing. They help us become aware of the unconscious polarities in our own psyches that we tend to deny or have difficulty accepting and dealing with. Healing occurs in partnership because we are mirrors to each other.

We need honest, loving, respectful feedback from partners to be able to grow. Everyone needs a partner equal to his or her own potential to evolve. Ask for spirit guidance in finding such an equal partner who is courageous enough to support your growth—in the same way you will support his or her growth. Partnerships are complex. We have to know who we are and select a partner who is up to the spiritual challenge of equally participating in accountability to grow. No compromise accepted. A true partner has the courage to hold the other accountable for change as they do themselves.

I often hear women and men voice their disappointment with their intimate partners. How does your partner's behavior symbolize your own? You might not want to know that answer but ask the question anyway. Ask yourself what your partner reflects about your childhood wound or the parts of you that you deny exist? Maybe it is time to deal with this particular issue in you. What are the partnership choices you need to make as part of your healing journey?

A stalemate partnership does not support growth and healing. An emotional conflict cycle in a deadlocked partnership may only encourage more wounds or staying in the old ones. Be honest and accountable. Identify and understand the destructive cycle and how you personally contribute and perpetuate that cycle in your partnership. Take a stand for your own growth. It may challenge your partner to be equally honest and accountable. One person is never responsible or capable of changing a destructive and wounding cycle on his or her own. When both partners are willing to see their own contribution to the trapping emotional cycle and each change their actions simultaneously, the relationship changes and heals.

A word of caution: insight about a negative cycle with a partner and even the ability to stop that cycle on occasion does not necessarily eliminate that cycle permanently. You may even leave the partnership and find that the negative cycle reoccurs in a slightly different but similar way in a new partnership. The other person does not bring the cycle into your life—you do.

Everyone needs the benefit of the doubt and an opportunity to repair his or her mistakes, but there is a limit. We need to confront loss and separation as a necessary price in the process of honest development if we want to achieve a true committed partnership in a progressing life.

Once your wounded theme reveals itself in a repetitive cycle, it reoccurs repeatedly in various ways to challenge you to grow and heal. Stay the course of your awareness and practice observation. Make sure that you move forward and not backward or sideways. The release from destructive or lifeless relationships will only occur when you are prepared to collaborate consciously with someone who will support and move proactively and willingly toward change and healing of themselves—as well as with you.

The most significant partner in your own psychic life is your body. Pay close attention to how your body reveals your hidden wounds and the way it keeps these in the cells of your organs. Release these aches and pains through bodywork, healthy eating, rest, and appropriate exercise. Take full ownership of—and attend to—your body. Your body also signals your soul's truth to you with sensations of peace and joy. Your body knows what is good for you and what is bad.

Know When to Say Yes and When to Say No

We always have a choice. Exercise the right to choose the options that serves your souls truth in any moment. Exercise your choice about when to engage and participate and when to exit conflict for instance. Exercise a choice about your beliefs and ideas. Know when it is a beginning of experiences, and when it is the end of a phase, conversation, or relationship. Despite the pull of our needs, fears, and desires, we always have a choice to act according to our soul-spirits truths. Say yes to what is right and no to what is not as your body and soul indicates.

The most difficult, challenging, and rewarding step in healing is to assert your truth. We liberate ourselves from repetitive emotional behavior when we act according to our truths. This liberating action happens because of a choice, and it usually opposes the pull from our personality's reactive responses.

Saying no implies a risk of losing the ones who are not pleased with our assertions. We may have to separate from these people. Separation implies loss, which we want to avoid, but our willingness to let go of what we thought we had to hold onto may be an essential aspect to our growth. Our growth necessitates leaving behind the people, places, and influences that no longer support our development. We separate from our mothers to go to school; we separate from our families to get married; we separate from our companies to collaborate with firms that support our careers better, and so on. Psychologically, we separate from one stage of life to a mature other.

Our willingness to separate from some people because of our choices to end destructive behavior patterns and emotional cycles at times is the right thing to do. We deceive ourselves when we suppress our truth—and this behavior can never protect the emotions of others. Letting yourself down will always let others down too—even if they tell you differently. Don't let your guilt responsibility for others and obligations deceive you.

Always base your choices on your truth. Your truth is always right for you as well as the people you leave. The choices we make to benefit our own truth become an opportunity for their growth too.

We also have to say no to destructive ideas and thoughts. We need to allow the mother of our outdated points of views to die in order to transform old belief structures into new life.

Know that God-You Is the Only Authority

I was presenting a paper on archetypes for a second time at a psychology conference. An elderly man eagerly introduced himself and told me how he still remembered and appreciated my previous presentation. He shared his despair over losing his driver's license that morning because of glaucoma. He asked what I thought the symbolic significance of this occurrence was. To him, this event was the most impactful trauma of his entire life since his only pleasure in life was driving. Speechless for a moment, I pondered how to respond to his emotional appeal.

It felt as if he had adorned me with the authority to present him with a significant answer that would clarify and improve his life. I fumbled under the weight of the responsibility. Tempted to rationalize the obvious, my first thought was that not having a motor vehicle urged him to find a new way to travel—also travel metaphorically.

A strange inner caution warned me about the obligation to supply a meaningful answer. Taking responsibility for solving this riddle might interfere with a sacred task that belonged to him alone. I reassured him that if he asked his inner self the question, the answer would be forthcoming. All he needed to do was stay alert and receptive; understanding would transpire in one form or other. We wished each other well and went our separate ways.

The meeting room was still empty when I arrived at the following presentation. Amazed, I found the same man asking for advice from the next presenter. He seemed to put more value on others' insight than his own, and I wondered why he negated his own inner wisdom.

A flash of understanding woke me up from a deep sleep that night. The man's driver's license was a symbol of independence and inner authority that he lost—he lost control over his life. The revocation of his license symbolized the loss of his inner power. He gave the responsibility of active self-determination to others and lost autonomy in his life journey. He became helpless. His dependency on others' guidance had put God on the outside of him rather than the inside.

The next morning, I told him that he had triggered an insight for me. Because there was no time to talk, I scribbled a metaphor on a piece of paper.

> And the man said, *"I do not have authorization to continue my life journey. This is the worst possible thing that can happen to my spirit. I lost my independence because I stopped exercising my power of vision. I assumed I am blind and rely on others to guide me."*

> And the angel in the man's soul said to him, *"Learn now and see clearly. Truth is in you. See where your power and your vision lie. Who controls the vehicle of your soul, and who steers the wheels of your destiny?"*

> And the man said, *"Oh, I see! For a moment, I looked away and lost myself. I am the true center of control. I accept my truth and my power."*

The incident with this man at the conference emphasized the importance that no other human or any of the identities our inner states of our egos identifies with have authority over us. Claim yourself, your body, mind, and soul. Convention, society, or others do not know the truth that applies to you. The truth is inside you. Your truth is not someone else's truth—and theirs not yours. God in you is the only authority ever to consider. People can mirror truth to you, but only your unique spiritual insight brings healing. We do not have authority over anyone. Our egos are not God over us or anyone else—and no one has any authority over you.

Someone else's truth may sound similar to your own when you have the same wound, but even so, you need to find your individual answer to your healing from your God-self.

Ask Questions

Ask yourself the difficult questions. Find answers you never expect to find by waiting patiently for your soul-spirit to reveal what you need to know regarding the questions. Our defense mechanisms mostly deceive us when we rely on our subjective side for answers. Ask your internal source of truth for guidance and clarity that supports your personality in its growth during every challenging circumstance.

I was once disappointed in a friend who lied to me. Whatever disturbs me in another person is a shadow part of myself that I need to know about. I denied that I was capable of lying so I asked my God-self what part of me was capable of lying. I waited patiently for an answer until I forgot that I asked the question. Then to my surprise, I observed myself—with amusement from my God-self—vastly exaggerating the facts of my story in a conversation with someone I needed to impress. There was my answer! I was unaware of my capacity to stretch the truth before that moment. My question gave me true insight into myself and also compassion for my friend who disappointed me so greatly. My consciousness about my fallibility also gave me a choice about my future behavior instead of unconsciously repeating behavior no one benefited from.

We get exactly what we need when we ask. Ask for awareness, understanding, and opportunities to learn and become aware. Ask for healing, love, acceptance, and courage. Ask your soul-spirit to inform you; your logical mind cooperating with your God-self.

Ask the right questions. Ask to know what part of you is talking to you and telling your how to interpret your perceptions. Ask what a particular fear is all about? Ask what a particular need is all about? Ask where in your life that particular ego-part originated? Ask how that ego-state relates to your ancestral wounds and your family or personal history? Ask yourself what defense mechanism your personality favors during challenges? Ask yourself what your soul-spirit wants your personality to learn through a particular challenge? Ask yourself what the healing response is to a particular challenge?

Formulating the right questions helps us focus the direction we take in our responses to challenges. Our ego-states easily misguide us. Questioning ourselves to get clarity about our fears, hopes, and ideals keeps us connected to the truth about our motivations and responses to life. Distinguish between the answers from your spirit and the answers from your personality.

Ask what your soul's purpose is right now? What is the theme of your current healing process, and how do your physical circumstances reflect that theme?

Ask advice from informed and wise experts, but let their guidance and support lead you to find your own truth. Be accountable in finding your true souls way, and do not rely on someone else to do the work for you. Our physical world changes according to our spiritual development and not the other way round.

Knowledge, experience, and information are tools to get to the truth— not truth itself. The truth is within us. Contemplate the meaning of something until the truth reveals itself instead of believing your first glance assumptions. Listen intensely to our soul-spirit by observing the non-verbal messages in daily life, synchronicities, metaphors, and symbols. Remember that our egos easily trick us. Make sure your insight comes from your soul-spirit by asking for confirmation of the insight; wait until clarity diminishes all doubt before you act on your insight. Our egos give us what we hope and wish for, or fear to hear and know. Our soul-spirits give us neutral realizations that resonates true, however scary to do. However, our egos will sometimes resist accepting these realizations and try to rationalize us away from our truth.

Get To Know the Archetypes

We use a map and guidebook to help us with relevant information about unfamiliar places on our travels. The Global Positioning System also makes our life easier by directing our movement from one place to another on earth. Without these tools, we might be lost—and our travel experiences will be less successful and enjoyable.

The universe functions and develops, according to principles of the divine archetypes. These archetypes are the building blocks of life and evolution. The archetypes serve as a map of our spiritual development processes towards evolution and consciousness. They inform the deeper, underlying meaning of our experiences. They guide us to understand our evolution in healing and the qualities and processes we go through to grow.

We recognize the spiritual purpose of the particular challenges we experience in life through recognizing the symbolic archetypal theme the experience represents. Our spiritual-emotional journey is far more exiting when we know where we are on this archetypal map and where we are going and why. Chapter 6 deals with the question of how to recognize the qualities and processes of the different archetypes and how to recognize a particular archetype during a particular personal circumstance. No archetype is more important or less important than any other. The diverse archetypes operate as one whole system with their unique but interrelated qualities. Wherever we are on this archetypal developmental map, we need to be there to participate in growth; exclusive as well as collective.

Dance between Opposites toward Wholeness

We gain balance by losing it. We learn about the existence of aspects of life through our subjective experiences that are usually one-sided viewpoints. As we realize that any emotional or other kind of experience reflects only one side of a polarity in our dualistic minds, we can immediately remind ourselves about the potential contrasting aspect that exists simultaneously. Bringing the contrasting element that opposes our experience into consciousness, we hold awareness of opposites as legitimate potentials in us. Through the back-and-forth movement of our attention between polarities, we get a glimpse of the simultaneousness of their existence which maintains balance in us because of this awareness.

Balance gives us a sense of neutral and objective peace and perfection because of our consciousness of opposites. Balance implies finding the point of stillness through a constant conscious movement between our opposite extremes. It is a readiness to experience an objective spiritual truth within the chaos of emotional entanglement and cognitive rationalizations. There is perfect order in the seeming chaos of life.

We wake up to balance between the wisdom of our soul-spirits and the pitfalls of our personalities through patient practice. We practice consciousness by moving between the opposite dimensions of our spiritual and our secular qualities. We practice consciousness by moving between the opposite dimensions of different daily activities.

Our breathing is a good example of achieving balance through awareness of opposites. Instead of breathing unconsciously, focus on how the inhale fills us up with vital oxygen that relaxes and nurtures every cell of our being with vital energy and recovery. Energy fuels our activities as we release the air on the outbreath. Our bodies act and our will exerts with every outbreath. There is a still point of perfect balance that happens between the inward and outward movements of air during breathing.

When we hold our breath during any activity, we get exhausted because we use willpower alone to fuel the activity and not the vital fuel of life we find in oxygen and life force. Breath is the symbol of life force. We use divine life force to act instead of ego power when we synchronize the connection between our egos and our God-selves. Consciousness enhances the deliberate balancing of these opposite—yet equally important—passive and active functions.

In the same way, we practice consciousness by allowing a still point of balance between work and play, family and profession, internal and external focus, and attention to body, mind, and spirit. Balance, however, is not a constant state; if it were, we would be stagnant. Balance continues to unfold though our experiences of imbalance. Allow the joy in that discovery and dance with it.

Share and Witness Stories of Growth

Take a stand for your truth. Stand firm and move confidently through life. Do not hide yourself; there is no shame in truth. Talk to others about the mysteries and wonders in your life when they are interested. Share your experiences with an attitude of objective wonder and gratitude; listen to others' experiences with appreciation. Keep an open mind to the creative possibilities of evolution without losing yourself. Be a loving and supportive witness to your own and others' spiritual development.

CHAPTER 6

Conceptual Model of the Meaning and Purpose of Life

What makes life meaningful? We generally equate meaning with happiness—and happiness with not having any problems. In an attempt to be happy, we try to avoid complications, but the harder we try to find a life without difficulties, the less we find that life. Our difficulties must have purpose and meaning too otherwise why do they exist?

Reality is never what it seems to be on first impact. When we think our life is problematic, those problems turns out to be the impetus for deliverance. When we think our life is happy, the happiness lulls us into stagnancy. Our collective unconscious motivates a deeper truth in our experiences than what our rational minds initially interpret. Our challenges provoke experiences, to wake us from our spiritual sleep. The conscious recognition of archetypal themes in our challenging encounters, provoked by our collective unconscious, brings purpose, significance, growth and healing once we decipher their underlying spiritual messages.

Our awareness moves beyond its initial ego-sensitized limitations. Meaning lies in the true purpose of why we are on the earth; it lies in growth and healing through awareness and choice.

Understanding Duality

A neuro-anatomist, Jill Bolte Taylor, wrote a personal account of her experience of suffering a massive stroke in her left hemisphere. Plume

Books published *My Stroke of Insight: A Brain Scientist's Personal Journey*, in May 27, 2009. She had little interest or awareness of her right hemisphere until this stroke.

Jill's identity as a scientist—and as an individual—diminished completely when her rational faculties, primarily situated in the left hemisphere, were not functioning. Her awareness of and familiarity with her daily responsibilities and stressors diminished completely. She was unable to speak or understand language; because of this, she only experienced life from a right-hemispheric perspective.

Her right hemisphere registered stimuli without her being able to interpret these perceptions. For Jill, there was no sense of separation between the rational and holistic realities of life any longer. Her awareness expanded into what she described as "bliss" and being one with all. She experienced herself as a pure energy being. Everything existed simultaneously. Because of the extreme circumstances of her brain damage, Jill was not aware of any boundaries and, therefore, had no individual identity. She intensely experienced unconditional love. She was only capable of sensing this love when her rational mind was unable to interfere and sensor these perceptions from the collective with rational interpretations.

Jill's story is an unusual and extreme example that does not instruct us to live in only a logical or only the collective unconscious mind, but it allows the promise of awareness and cooperation between these faculties. Jill's experience leaves us with a clearer concept of the possibilities of our non-verbal collective intelligence.

The complementary hemispheres of our brain are one example of the amazingly complex complementary system of our physical, emotional, and spiritual vehicle as a whole. Objective and subjective reality converge continually in our physical body. This is where our personalities and soul-spirits merge, where heaven and earth, past and future becomes the sacred present.

Table 1 may help to illustrate the differences between left-brain and right-brain functions, but it is not an absolute parameter. Always remember that our hemispheres are complementary and rely upon each other. In reality, they work together for an undivided, complementary "whole."

Left-Hemisphere Functions	Right-Hemisphere Functions
Factual	Intuitive
Sequential	Parallel
Planned	Random
Rational	Holistic
Analytical	Synthesizing
Looks at Parts	Experiences the Whole
Verbal	Symbolic
Quantitative	Qualitative
Organized	Synchronized
Individualized	Interpersonal
Specific	Collective
Interpretative	Kinesthetic

Table 1 Left- and Right-Hemisphere Functions

Our bodies are vehicles for the creative expression of the primary divine archetypal themes, the building blocks of life that guide us during our unfolding life. The dualistic nature of our ego-driven personalities connects with our God-potentials inside our bodies to access divine revelations through subjective experiences. When we open ourselves to the objective reality through our right hemispheres, insight and illumination are spontaneous.

Together, logic and objective spiritual illumination equals insight that allows creative growth and healing. The belief that our rational minds alone are objective is false. Most of the time, we are unaware of just how subjective we are because of our ignorance of our defensive conditioned personal unconscious. Take a moment to become familiar with the right- and left-hemispheric faculties. Practice awareness of where and how these abilities operate in your life. Make space for your right hemisphere to partake in your experiences as much as you allow your left hemisphere that privilege. Acknowledging these different faculties and practicing the distinction between their operations help us know ourselves better.

Life evolves according to archetypal principles. We connect with these archetypes in the collective unconscious. We connect with the collective unconscious through our bodies, our non-verbal senses, our intuition, synchronicities and dreams. Our non-verbal nature uses the language of metaphor and symbol to communicate its truths. Our individual ego-identities have no influence on the collective unconscious. Objective truth has no agenda. The objective truth we find in the collective unconscious carries no fear, need for survival, or desire.

Objective truth is about eternal collective principles that promote life itself in creative dynamic processes toward healing and wholeness. We recognize the principles of objective truth in symbols and metaphors we find in our subjective experiences. Human nature is a complex multidimensional system. Understanding how we interrelate and connect to all the aspects of our being is essential.

Figure 1 illustrates the range of human faculties, each with its particular comprehensive systems that function in the most concrete forms to the most abstract of principles. Our physical bodies orchestrate all of our possible senses and awareness's in a physical form that we maintain and operate from on the earth. Our physical body serves as our spiritual vehicle that integrates all that we are. Our spiritual life expresses itself through our physical nature once we connect with it. Our energetic body orchestrates the electric and magnetic neural activity of our nervous system. Our mental body orchestrates our mind, thoughts, beliefs, and attitudes. Our brain is the place of mental operations. Our brain is a dual hemispheric organ with an ability to register the dimensions of both rational-verbal and intuitive non-verbal. Together, the mental, energetic, and physical bodies form the emotional body, which regulates our subjective reality through our personalities with its ego-states. Our ego-states create the emotional repetitive conflict cycles that maintains our status quo.

Our subjective reality is predominantly determined by the functions of our left hemisphere, and our intuitive reality operates beyond the realm of rational mind and language. The intuitive body, or faculty, bridges the capacities of the creative right hemisphere and the rational left hemisphere. All our faculties work together to access and process both the subjective as well as the objective realities into insight. Accessing the collective objective reality into all that is our physical vehicle, we wake up to operating as the aware and evolving being that we are.

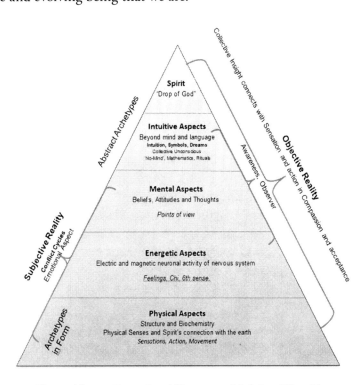

Figure 1 Inter-dimensional Human and Spiritual Faculties

This kind of mental alertness, yet stillness, implies a collective spiritual consciousness that leads to our healing. The objective reality we are talking about in this particular context is the un-manifested divine potential or love-consciousness (Christ-consciousness) that permeates existence itself.

Christ consciousness is the knowing that God is in every human being and is accessed through the collective unconscious. This is where the building blocks of life—the core archetypes—manifest their purest creative God-essence which we all have in us. The collective unconscious wakes us up to consciousness of our connection to our divine nature.

The Anatomy of Archetypes

The universe functions according to the principles of core archetypes. Archetypes are the building blocks that direct all of life dynamically and creatively. These principles shape our human experience and evolution.

Archetypes remain constant in their fundamental meaning and potential as they organize themselves in a dynamic variety of human expressions potentials and experiences. The timeless themes of these principles reveal deeper psychological and cosmological meanings that give form, order, and development to our lives. Our defensive egos interpret the challenges our unconsciousness manifests in secular life as painful struggles and liberates ourselves from this idea as we learn to solve the mysteries of the archetypal messages.

We cannot separate ourselves from the archetypes—we can only move along with their series of unfolding themes as we progress in our development with the rest of creation throughout and beyond time. We acquire firsthand, intimate comprehension of the universal substances and characteristics as we recognize our subjective experiences as symbolic communications from our spirit, informing us about purpose. It is helpful to our psychological and spiritual development to understand how we relate to and develop according to the challenges that correspond to these archetypal principles.

Personality Types and Archetypal Themes

Core archetypes are the primary elements of the creative living universe. These symbolic themes present in our experiences express the creative qualities and principles of the archetypes. Our subjective experiences mirror these archetypes but are not the essences of the archetypes themselves. An archetypal energy expresses its creative potential as a polarized range of possibilities in our subjective personality. Each archetype holds constructive and destructive potential in our human expression.

There are many possible expressions of the archetypal themes along a continuum of positive and negative possibilities. The human ego identifies with particular parts in the range of possibilities, drawing us into those particular patterns of subjective expressions, and we recognize them in our behavior over time. The quality we identify with allows subjective feelings that legitimize our identity.

We judge the qualities we adhere to as either good or bad. We perceive life through the particular viewpoint of the qualities we identify with—as if no other exists—and we forget that we connect to all the archetypes and contain them all within us. Our subjective selves do not like the idea of our capacity for both good and bad.

Expanded awareness opens us to all the possibilities as a potentiality, which gives us conscious choice over our behavior. Our unconsciousness of our positive and negative potential keeps us fallible and deluded about who we are. We do not have to consent to hurtful or negative behavior, but we need to accept it as part of our human nature. The polarity of good and bad becomes a circular concept that eliminates judgment. The whole contains all opposites. Opposites are complementary and reflect the latent opposite side within itself. Each side of a polarity is never an absolute state; they both belong together, and the one leads to the other. Our knowledge of our full abilities develops liberation from compulsive reactions and helps us cultivate compassion and choice, enabling change and growth.

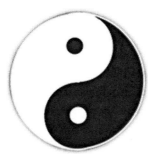

Figure 2 Yin-Yang Symbol

The yin-yang symbol in Figure 2, drawn from Chinese dualistic philosophy, demonstrates the polarity of positive and negative qualities within life. Opposites complete each other in a contained circle, the symbol of the whole. The same principle applies to every archetypal theme. There are two extremes, seemingly disconnected, yet interconnected and interdependent, just as the seasons in the natural world give rise to each other in turn. Winter becomes summer, and summer becomes winter. Night becomes day, and day becomes night. Each seemingly polarized aspect contains the essence of and complements the other. Birth becomes death, and death becomes birth. The negative teaches us the good, and the good teaches us the negative.

Suzette (a fictional name for a client) sought help for her tendency to compromise her needs by ignoring her inner promptings. Let us consider

Suzette's struggle to find the right partner as an example to illustrate the concept of identifying the constructive and destructive perspectives of her circumstances. She allows herself to start relationships with men who are obviously wrong for her. As a result, she continually feels worthless when these relationships break up. She tolerates wrong choices and her subsequent unhappiness for fear of disappointing others' ideas about who she should be with and accept. She is a pleaser and does not listen to her own inner voice.

Suzette believes that she will be alone for the rest of her life if she does not accept the first man who shows interest in her. She is more conscious of her fear and gives her fear priority over her inner voice. An ego-state with an agenda to be in a relationship that would give her value regardless drives this fear and becomes a repetitive pattern of disillusionment and inauthentic relationships. Her ego-state is ruling her rational mind to the extent that she is too fearful to change her behavior. The repetitive pattern confirms Suzette's belief that her challenge in her dilemma means that she is unworthy of having a partner.

Her father left her mother for another woman, and Suzette internalizes the sense that she too is not good enough for love. Her passive submission and suppression of her needs is a defense mechanism. The constructive potential of her psyche lies in her choice to do the opposite of her defensive action. Her acceptance of loneliness and independence as a reality while she acknowledges the true qualities she needs in a partner, without compromising, will attract her true partner to her.

The constructive aspects of our dilemma seems the most difficult to act on, but in reality the destructive aspects of our dilemma is the behavior that hurts us most and we find easiest to repeat. Now let us consider the constructive and destructive aspects of all the archetypes.

Examples of the Psychological Defense-Mechanisms as They Connect to the Personality's Interpretations of the Archetypes

The Multi-Dimensional Idealist

This archetype is about the morals and principles that secure healthy development and evolution in the universe. It is about recognizing the right action that promotes healthy life as a multidimensional being in a multidimensional universe. It is also about the recognition and respect of all life as we participate in evolution—on all the levels of existence—with our ability to use and promote the creative forces of all the elements in creation.

Our personality, prior to spiritual awareness, tries to do the right thing. We honor morality, principles, willpower, and a focused mind with a conscience. The defense mechanism the personality applies to this archetypal awareness is a "reaction formation" where one blocks desire by its opposite emotion to avoid anger from self or others when one fails to apply high morals and principles. The personality can become moralistic and dogmatic, and it desires acknowledgment of its righteousness.

We may be idealistic workaholics or judgmental perfectionists when we identify with this archetype. We may inspire others to improve and protect a healthy life and development because of our natural insight of universal laws and principles. We may show good judgment and leadership. This personality struggles with a fear of being bad or wrong. The pathology associated with this defense mechanism is obsessive-compulsive behavior.

The Healing Process of the the Multi-Dimensional Idealist

To be human is to learn about perfection by moving between all the dimensions and our abilities. Magic happens when we acknowledge our multidimensionality as well as how we hold the multitude of dimensions, together with others, as we continue to develop. We recognize and regard the higher principles of universal cycles and laws, the bigger picture that directs life. We can take people in and accept all others as equals at the soul level. We can be open to the flow of energy from the source of creation with all its aspects. The top of the throat is the location in our bodies that relate to this archetype. Our awareness of this archetypal energy center can bring us closer to engaging in a relationship with the source of creation to affirm that all life is spiritual and sacred.

The Connector

This archetype is about promoting connection and communication between all aspects of life in the universe, through service. It is about a compassionate awareness of emotions and truth and the collaboration and cooperation between all people. It is about generously serving and helping to support all beings with understanding and connecting with love. It is about repairing connections through intuitive awareness of others' needs and feelings.

The defense mechanism that the personality applies under the influence of this archetype is repression. When we suppress and disregard our instinctual impulses, we repress. Our personalities suffer fear of others not being able—or wanting—to love us. The pathology associated with this defense mechanism in the personality is *passive aggressive and passive abusive behavior.*

The Healing Process of the Connector

Engagement means that we move between the parts involved. The back-and-forth interaction and negotiation between the needs of others and our own needs balances and repairs disconnection. When we connect and interact joyfully with everyone around us—and with all the aspects of ourselves—we find common ground to balance. Engaging with our complementary aspects in others helps us all to evolve creativity in and through all our relationships. The solar plexus is the body zone that connects with this archetype and registers an internal vibration that makes it easy for us to receive and respond to others energies.

The Performer

This archetype is about productivity and development. It is about producing through the principle of beauty and love in the secular reality that serves all beings on spiritual and physical levels. The faculty of creative imagination manifests by being completely present in our body in every moment. This archetype teaches us the importance of manifesting spirit in our bodies.

The defense mechanism used here is identification. When we emulate another by identifying with their ideals of success and status, we identify with those and take them as our own. We focus on becoming or pretending to be what we think our role models expect from us. We focus on impressing others with our talents and achievements because of the idea that those qualities we admire and emulate will have others admire us too. When our personalities unconsciously model who we think we should be on another's ideals, we fear disappointment and try to avoid failure at all costs. Seeking status and wanting to be admired above all else our personalities become ambitious, competitive, or dishonest and we hide our true feelings. The fear of not having value is paramount to us. The pathology associated with this defense mechanism of identification in the personality is martyrdom and narcissism.

The Healing Process of the Performer

Imagination that turns dreams into inspiration ends all pretentiousness. Our true abilities unfold when our unique potentials shape into inspirational qualities that inspire others. We consider ourselves as equal participants that move toward a cooperative future. This archetype relates to the top of the sternum in our bodies from where we can focus on the spiritual essence of our unique soul qualities.

The Champion

This archetype is about protecting the principle of creative life force in all others by manifesting and preserving this power of life through giving structure, direction, order, and directing creative action from our hearts, heads, and spirits.

Introjection is the defense mechanism of the personality when it relates to this archetype. This means that we have a personal expectation of ourselves to take responsibility for others. Our personalities carry the burdens of holding ideals, ideas, objects, processes, and people in direct and organized care. Intense responsibility alleviates the feeling of insignificance. We fear loss of significance and connection with the people, ideas, and objects we feel responsible to. The pathology associated with this defense mechanism is a dependent or co-dependent personality as well as depression.

The Healing Process of the Champion

We have to align ourselves completely with our own life and not another. We have to take our place firmly and commit to live in our own body, mind, and soul. We have to take our personal place in the universe with an internal sense of our own nature, our own right to be here, and our own authority. Our committed presence in ourselves allows us to feel a sense of our own significance. Our worthiness does not depend on others feeling protected by us. We do not need to be a hero. This archetype relates to the lower abdomen in our bodies that sense emotion intensely. Release all the emotions you carry for others from this area.

The Observer

This archetype is about contemplation and the principles of learning and teaching. It is about accessing knowledge through sensitive objective observation—not only through logic but also by listening to clarifications from sources beyond the known. Humanity progresses in its current understanding through new understandings that transcend the current ones. Focus and concentration are required to witness understanding, meaning, and wisdom. This archetype generates the energy of the scientist.

When we associate with this archetype, our personalities use the defense mechanism of isolation. It is about distancing and disconnection from others by retreating from life and the world in order to dedicate all our energy to find meaning beyond the status quo. The personality fears meaninglessness, emptiness, and incapability. When we get lost in the fears of this archetype we do feel empty and disconnected. The pathology associated with this defense mechanism is the schizoid personality and schizophrenia.

The Healing Process of the Observer

Connect with others in organizations or disciplines. Work in groups to develop your trust in others and recognize new understanding and meaning in cooperation with them. Knowing and having an awareness of the big picture—the realization that everything in the universe is knowable—brings mental peace instead of futility. The crown of the head is the place in our bodies that relate to this archetype and where we find the energetic gateway to connect to this kind of contemplation that allows new understanding.

The Skeptic

This archetype is about solving the internal dilemma between loyalty and defiance through insight and love. We find the source of unconditional love, insight, and appreciation in our connection with the center of the earth, our mother. We make authentic choices by weighing the opposite possibilities until an outcome resonates with our heart's truth and our minds logic. The conflict between loyalty and defiance engage us in reason and love, which are both essential activities to determine balance and equilibrium. Fairness is born from ambivalence that stirs both faculties of our psyche.

Our personalities are devoted but cynical, ambivalent, yet dutiful. It is difficult to trust. The defense mechanism is projection. This personality blames and projects unwanted traits on others who become their scapegoats. The wounds of the skeptic are about security and trust. The skeptic defies loved ones or others because they suffer a fear of losing support and guidance. The extreme pathology associated with this defense mechanism is ambivalence and paranoia.

The Healing Process of the Skeptic

We discover that the fears we hold in ourselves make us see others in a negative light. We choose to commit to supporting others without our own fears pulling us into doubt. The center of our sternum is the place in our bodies that resonates with this archetype. This is where we sense the vibration of all things in life. This is the place in our bodies that like a drum is connected with the center of our being and to our earth roots. We focus on noticing the voice of truth in our hearts and balance more deeply by practicing rational discernment in our choices which help us accept life and people.

The Entrepreneur

This archetype is about the principle of mastering through change. It is about the ability to recognize stagnation and move beyond it with deliberate action toward growth and health. It is about thinking beyond the status quo that comes from accessing and connecting a variety of information in creative, insightful ways. Mastering is the ability to free ourselves from the traps of our limiting ideas by not acting from our humanness but from our divine source. While we do accept the fact that we are human, we practice to focus our thoughts on the point where we are divine mind to access this neglected faculty. Focus and concentration help us release all the unnecessary excess of conditioned ideas and fears that interferes with our understanding transformation and growth.

The personality uses the defense mechanism of rationalization with this archetype. The use of logic and reason justifies behavior in order to avoid pain and sorrow at all cost. When defensive, our personalities are only interested in avoiding hardship and go after the new and exciting distractions instead of making the changes needed for growth and healing. The personality that connects to this archetype fears confinement, pain, deprivation, and boredom. Pathology associated with this defense mechanism is the histrionic personality or hysteria and mania.

The Healing Process of the Entrepreneur

The entrepreneur can achieve mastery by reaching for a still point in the the mind. The still point is a neutral attitude where there is no thought. The mind is important to this archetype. The process of letting go of what we think we know sets us free to access information beyond the mind from the collective unconscious where there are infinite possibilities of new original insights. Eliminating old, rigid ideas opens up the ability to transition toward the unfolding of new possibilities. The center of the forehead or the third eye is the place in our bodies that can quiet our mind and bring us to that still point that transcends time and space where we access the truth we need to grow.

The Courageous

This archetype is about the principle of maintaining and developing courage, control, self-esteem, and personal integrity when challenged by the dark and destructive side of life. These destructive influences challenge us to learn about our inner strength and courage that helps us stand firm in our power to trust the reliability and creativity of the universe. Cherishing life despite hardship creates courage, strength, and trust.

The personality uses the defense mechanism of denial. We avoid owning up to our weaknesses or wrongdoings when we relate to this archetype. We may also deny our power and live with an impression of being a powerless victim against merciless life. Power is revered and weakness despised—or we internalize weakness and deny power. The personality fears others controlling and harming them, and we can become controlling, ruthless, and harmful or feel weak against external power. The personality exploits others and nature ruthlessly without regard for boundaries or only relates to nature and animals with no trust in humans. The pathology associated with this defense mechanism is anti-social or psychopathic behavior (acting without conscience).

The Healing Process of the Courageous

We develop integrity and self-respect by allowing ourselves to manage our boundaries, first in our bodies and then between us and others as well as the natural world and us. We respect and do not violate others' boundaries. At the same time, we honor ourselves and do not allow anyone to violate our boundaries. We learn to know how to turn an idea into a manifested reality that maintains harmony with others and nature.

Our power manifests to enhance all life and not harm humanity or nature. The base of the spine, the sacrum, is the place in the body that relates to this archetype. Our sacrum grounds us with a strong instinct to detect and protect all necessary boundaries—between nature and humanity and between others and us. Our firm and watchful awareness synchronizes the connection between our soul, our body, and the earth. We are dependable.

The Moderator

This archetype is about the principle of all-inclusiveness and the assimilation and conclusion of all learning. It is about introspection and negotiation for peace among all and the integration of all that we have ever encountered. Everyone and everything is included without judgment or conditions. We share our wisdom, experiences—and support healing and growth for all—as we evolve together through life.

The personality uses the defense mechanism of self-narcotization, which is a numbing of the self by escaping reality, especially the sense that we do not want to be in our physical body in a physical reality. All addictive behavior indicates this kind of escape mechanism. We distract ourselves from secular life with drugs, work, television, food, spirituality, or fantasy. The personality fears conflict. The pathology associated with this defense mechanism is evident in avoidant behavior or addictions.

The Healing Process of the Moderator

We assimilate all we know into a comprehensive whole and share it with others as we live our assimilated wisdom. The body assimilates all experiences into a comprehensive teaching through our breath. Our breath becomes an important mechanism to help us open up as we receive and exert energy. Breathing is our way of claiming life and accepting our physical destiny. Breathing is a practice of ongoing healing and transformation.

We continue to collect the pieces and parts of understanding and wisdom. Then we assimilate them in ways that heal ideas and emotions from the past. Healing is a process of completion, using our breath to find peace. The spot between our shoulder blades synchronizes the movement of our breath and lungs so that we can move into harmony and become one with the whole.

The Personality and Its Many Ego-States

"The single story creates stereotypes, and the problem with stereotypes is not that they are untrue, but that they are incomplete. They make one story become the only story."

—*Chimamanda Ngozi Adichie*

Our personality contains many ego-states (aspects of the ego) that resemble all the archetypal themes. Together the archetypes form one synchronized structure that maintains and continue to create life and we are made of the same stuff as the universe—in the image of God. Driven by fear and desires, our egos—with its assembly of different ego-states—modify the divine archetypes into personal schemas. Schemas are sets of ideas beliefs and actions motivated by specific fears and desire to reinforce those beliefs. Each ego-state reveals a specific fear-driven behavior based on beliefs and defensive emotional conditioning. Together, all our ego-states form the composition of our personalities which then influence our everyday reactive behavior with its fear-based defensive schematic arrangements unconsciously. Fear is the ultimate factor that challenges our biological and physical survival instincts. Our ego's task is to maintain our personality's survival instinct by confirming its schemas.

Because our ego-states drive our personalities unconsciously, we are helpless to the effect of these schemas until we realize how powerfully subjective our behavior is. We have no free choice as long as our point of view comes from the one-sidedness of any of our ego-states. The ego-interpreted impressions of our experiences keep us bonded in subjective perspective that distorts our reality. We feel incomplete, and we stay unaware of how our reactive responses maintain our subjectivity until we become aware of the collective unconscious. Awareness of the collective unconscious includes the faculties we need to complete our nature to be capable of objectivity.

To free ourselves from our own blindness, we need to know how the schemas of each of our ego-states influence our reactions. We also need to know how to connect to our spiritual nature and its potential in complementing our perceptions. The association we cultivate between our subjective cognitive as well as our collective unconscious unites our functioning into an objective creative evolving self. This self is our God-self where our humanness and God-side act as one integrated being.

Our ego-states with their specific schemas claim identities we recognize from our personality's point of view as the "me" or the "I". We say: "that is who I am or what I am". Our personalities identify with these characteristics but exclude all aspects that are not accepted by the ego but still present in our unconscious. Our ego parts are also not usually aware of our God-self unless we instruct it to become aware. Ego with all its parts only focuses on preserving the specific qualities it maintains as their identities to the exclusion of all else in the construct of our psyches. Our ego-states do not easily relinquish its position of control in our personalities. We therefore feel as if we have no power over these ego-state identities. The different ego-states even rally for positions to control one another inside our personalities. That is why some traits are stronger than others in us and they resist changing their point of view for another part in us to exercise influence in our choices. We become so convinced about these particular traits as our identity that they start to rein supremely over all the rest of our potential and latent qualities.

Together, all the conscious and unconscious ego-states or parts of our nature form our personality. When we say, "I feel this or think that," we are under the impression that we are talking from the center of our being. In fact, we are taking perspective from a specific point of view of one of the many ego-states that reside in our personality.

The ego-states take turns playing their emotional tunes or schemas through recognizable themes; they control our ideas, beliefs, and emotional reactions to life. Depending on the circumstances, we become playful, childlike, or responsible and goal-oriented. Different aspects of us take turns to drive our personality, fulfilling a variety of roles.

Some of our ego-states never get a turn and stay hidden in our personal unconscious. When any one of the many ego-states takes command inside our psyche, we are especially aware of an emotional compulsion that repeats a specific behavior associated with that particular ego-state schema. We emphasize the ego-states we strongly identify with and cultivate. We convince ourselves to accept or reject the traits we want and those we do not stay unconscious or suppressed but still present in our psyches. The unrecognized or suppressed ego-states in our personal unconscious become shadow-states. We react with intense emotion when we recognize these suppressed aspects of ourselves as shadow qualities in others. When we least expect it, our shadow behavior surprises and sometimes shock us. We exclaim, "That is not me!" I don't usually do that kind of thing?" "The words just came out of my mouth"

There are two contradicting forces in our psyche. On the one hand, we perceive and experience life through our subjective ego-oriented personality. Our personality and its ego-states focus on and drive us toward the individual, survival-based, socially conditioned ideas we identify with as ourselves. On the other hand, we perceive and experience a collective unconscious, not based on personal ambition or fear, but beyond the personal. This non-ego aspect is as much part of us as the other but completely neglected and sometimes rejected.

This collective unconscious side urges our spiritual development from an objective, transpersonal consciousness. These two realities operate simultaneously in our beings. Our awareness is mostly preoccupied with one reality at a time. We are aware of our subjective reality while the unconscious collective reality tries to reach our consciousness through signs, synchronicities, symbols, and symptoms. Our ego-states are most comfortable with the logical world of individual survival because this is what they understand best. We are out of practice, and we do not always know how to access the non-verbal, intuitive faculties that connect us to the collective transpersonal dimension. It is however necessary to integrate all the aspects of being inside us for the sake of our healing and evolution

The non-linear, subtle language of symbolism speaks to us without rational interpretations. By silencing personal efforts from our ego, we learn to receive and accept awareness from the objective reality. Without ego interference, insight integrates these dual worlds. Our rational mind accepts the gifts of the non-verbal world and comes to a more meaningful awareness than was previously possible.

The drop-of-God emerges as a creative energy within us that facilitates the bridge where our cognitive intelligence, physical body, and subjective and collective unconscious meet and integrate. This creative merging becomes the new self—our authentic truth, essence, and wholeness. This self-essence always urges healing of humanity and the individual. It is timeless and unconditional in its acceptance of what is in the moment, and it drives us toward the eternal universal. Our drop-of-God directs the orchestra of ego-states with acceptance and insight, and it gives us perspective on our ability to heal from emotional conflict cycles.

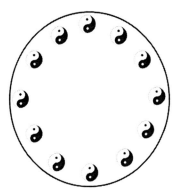

Figure 3 Personality with Many Ego-States

Figure 3 symbolizes the personality; its many ego-states together resemble the potential of the objective whole. Each ego-state develops its personalized schemas from our environmental influences by using the archetypal building blocks already present in us. The schemas are morphed impressions of the original archetypes—not the actual archetypes.

The figure further illustrates how some ego-states maintain a central position of control in our personality that colors our perspective with its own schema. This is why most of what we experience is subjective. Our personality is driven and is obliged to follow a few specific patterns of behavior, depending on the leading ego-state schemas in our personality. We identify with the specific ego-states that lead, compete, and assert against other suppressed ego-states.

Figure 4 demonstrates how a few ego-states can work together to sovereignly control our personality—or take turns in the driver's seat of our personality.

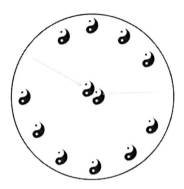

Figure 4 Personality with One or More Ruling Ego-States

Our task is to discover the true archetypal potential of our psyche and allow ourselves to develop all these qualities instead of cultivating the schemas that our personalities use to perpetuate our wounds. Our personalities should rather be employed in the service of our soul-sprit to express the original purpose of our divine potential than our shortsighted egos agendas. Our personalities focus on a limiting perspective of our soul-spirit's potential but once we free ourselves from our imagined limitations we understand our complete compilation of our faculty's qualities and potentialities. Our complete integration of the compilation of archetypes reassures our healing and wholeness. Honoring and respecting the meaning of divine differences enhances all of life. We can live a complementary, harmonious life.

Our subjective worldview limits us from being inclusive of all objective potential. However, the only way we learn about each archetype is to experience it subjectively within the context of our ego. Our egocentric personalities are necessary for our human experiences to inform us about our underlying spiritual understanding. It is from our subjective perspective that we open to transformation through the particular experiences of life when we reconnect with our divine collective nature. Our soul-spirits are creatively expressed in and through our personalities.

The Drop-of-God in Us

God is not a religion; God is our universal consciousness. God is us and not separate from us. We wake up to God-consciousness and incorporate it into our practical lives.

Our personalities fear life and take on the burden of coping with life alone without realizing we are connected to the universal spiritual inside us as a partner in evolution. It is difficult for our personalities to perceive or be conscious of all the facets of the universe at once. Our personalities perceive life therefore from a limiting perspective and cope with only a few—or one—subjective awareness at a time. Our subjective involvement has us focus on the singular instead of the multidimensional. Because we identify with only some qualities of life—and not all at once—we suffer a sense of separateness from our spiritual essence that connects us to our universal creative life force. The identities that our egos initially focus on are learning experiences that inform us of those particular qualities in the universe. We go through many experiences that we add together to eventually complete our picture of the whole within and how we fit in with all around us. As we add our accumulated experiences over time, our awareness about our full potential grows. We find that we are connected to all that exist and hold the potential of the whole within us even though we participate as individuals in our specific and unique learning experiences. We have the whole universe within us.

This transpersonal perspective is the creative drop-of-God we encounter as the full universal potential in us. The drop-of-God in us is the eternal life force that exists in us as it exists in all that exists. We make objective sense of experiences when the universal life force in us communicates through symbol from the non-verbal dimension to our accepting and receptive rational dimension. Our drop-of-God has no personal agenda; it is only interested in the truth of our experience as it applies to our healing. It allows us to release all subjective conflict with objective wisdom. The emerging drop-of-God infuses us with a capacity of whole-sighted love toward all that exists. We gain a perspective beyond our personal subjective and, in this way, develop authenticity with our true reality as a whole being.

We discover the drop-of-God in our psyches by listening patiently for the subtle language of the objective in synchronicities and symbols. God is in the details of subtle observation of these synchronicities, metaphors and symbols. Our personalities tend to ignore everything that is not ego-based and easily misses the messages from our soul-spirits. We need to be aware of the battle between our egos and our God-selves where our egos try to suppress our God-selves because it preserves this part as a threat to its sovereign survival. Our personalities try to preserve its ego-selves competitively with defense mechanisms that overrule the subtle teachings of the objective. Sometimes, we only heed the messages of our drop-of-God side when trauma renders our ego-defenses incapable and we become humble and willing to surrender to our God-side's insight and guidance.

Life is a creative process that requires constant receptivity, observation, evaluation, reorientation, application, and adjustment of our insights through choice. Objective awareness is only possible when our personality employs our God-self as described above.

Our drop-of-God becomes the true "I" when our identity actively includes our soul-spirit parts into our personalities above the close-minded agendas of our ego-states. Our God-self collaborates with our subjective personality in becoming a whole person; the essential Self at the center of our being as illustrated in Figure 5. It is our God-selves that are capable of unconditional love for our ego states and guide us to not succumb to the pressure of ego agendas. Real choices are possible when we live in this awareness. Our ego states are no longer the rulers of our personalities but on the periphery of what is now our whole psyche. As a whole integrated being we love our ego states with awareness and compassion as we experience life through their eyes but no longer feel trapped by their emotional interpretations. Our God-selves direct the union of all the ego sides with objectivity.

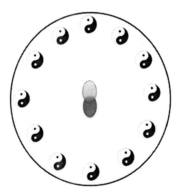

Figure 5 God-Self Felt as the Drop-of-God

Repetitive Conflict Cycles

A conflict cycle is a pattern of behavior based on false beliefs and ideas that motivate our personalities about how to gain self-worth. Our culture and families usually condition us to believe these ideas, which become our ego-state parts with their schemas which forms our personalities.

Fears fuel specific ideas that promote defenses against the loss of what our ego-states believe will secure self-worth. This internal psychological arrangement forms an unconscious repetitive cycle of ideas, perception, emotions, and reactive behavior.

Initially our ego believes that its unconscious defense mechanisms protect our existence and identity; it is a survival instinct. As we mature, these defenses become redundant as we realize that we perceive our world according to the triggers that set off these defense mechanisms. We keep on repeating them and don't know how to get out of the trap of the cycles we created. Staying in the repetitive conflict cycle stunts our growth and healing and keeps us wounded by us holding on to the wounds that started the defensive cycle in the first place. Once we are aware of our instinctive behavior cycles, we learn to exercise choice over our responses by distinguishing between our ego's training and our essential worthiness.

We find liberation once we move beyond our defensive repetitions by responding to life with a clear perception and complete acceptance of objective reality as it is—and not as our wounds have conditioned us to assume and our emotional agendas have us react. We can understand our own behavior cycles by observing the symptoms we experience and then track our emotions embedded in the symptoms to the origin of the wounds that started the defensive mechanisms.

The cycle that traps us usually indicates a clear fear-need theme that is explicit to a specific ego-state. The particular fear-need theme of an ego-state always colors our experience with emotionally subjective perceptions. We perceive all occurrences through lenses of a particular theme until we become conscious of our ego-states and the origin of their wounds. These conflict-filled themes unconsciously repeat over many generations in a variety of ways. Our personal, family, and cultural histories clearly portray these reoccurring emotional conflict themes. We identify the common internal and interpersonal conflict patterns by the particular fears, thoughts, defense mechanisms, and emotions that manifest in our reoccurring behavior.

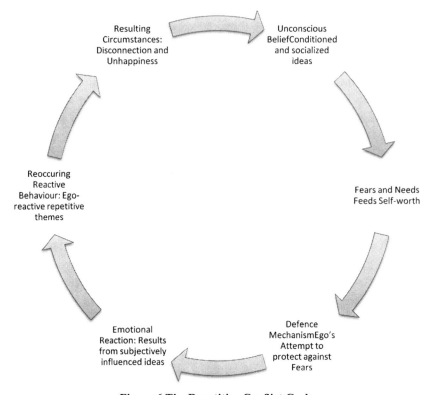

Figure 6 The Repetitive Conflict Cycle

Figure 6 illustrates the repetitive conflict cycle as a closed circle, moving in a particular reactive arrangement, driven by a themed emotion, fear, unconscious defense mechanism, conscious belief, and reactive behavior pattern. It is easy to analyze how the pattern occurs in our personal life and understand how the theme came about by analyzing our history.

An example of one such a behavior pattern occurs for instance in the scenario of someone who has a compulsion to do things right and be right. Perfectionism is the persistent quality for this person that provides meaning, purpose, and self-worth, but it also drives the primary fear of being wrong, bad, or imperfect. The person striving to be perfect becomes obsessive-compulsive. They feel singularly responsible to fix the world and everybody in it. To be imperfect would mean that they are unworthy and incomplete. They project this theme of the need to be perfect on others too.

We judge behavior according to our subjective perceptions, colored by our fears and needs. A vicious cycle sets in motion when our willpower feeds the desire to be perfect because of the fear to lose value by not being good enough. Perfectionism can create anxiety, anger, attempts to control and judge. Entanglement in this conflict cycle feeds our discontentment with life and ourselves. It results in unhappiness and disconnection with others. We may actually escalate the conflict cycles we engage in by staying unconscious of our desires and fear-driven motivators.

In reality, each of the core archetypes with their specific themes holds a key for our transformation and is, in contrast to the subjective expressions of them, completely neutral. They have no agenda for self-worth. Worthiness is undisputed and cannot be earned in any way. Life is about experiences for growing consciousness not earning worthiness. It is only our ego-states with their socially conditioned agendas that provoke false beliefs in our personalities of generating unworthiness upon neglect of perusing the trained agendas. Objective perception of conflict cycles illuminates our closed-circuit behavior patterns to reveal the answers for our healing.

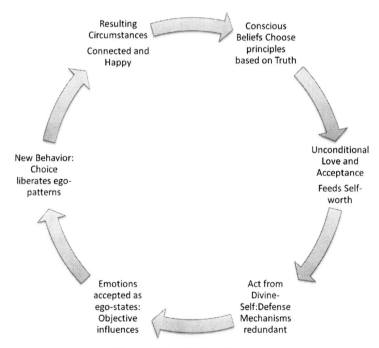

Figure 7 The Healing Response

The healing response pattern illustrated in Figure 7 identifies our egos struggles and, in contrast to these conditioned patterns, chooses to act from our spiritual perspectives. Healing is a process where we practice acting in a direction counter to the driving force of the ego. When we give in to the driving force of the ego, we repeat the cycle, so we have to turn around from the cycle by going in the opposite direction. We are able to choose change and healing by moving opposite to the pull of our conditioning. In the case of perfectionism, we allow ourselves to correct our mistakes and grow because of the experience.

Our egos find it difficult to believe that it can be unconditionally accepted and be worthy without having to prove worthiness. Our egos attempt to prove its identity by believing to be the subjective hero that controls all of life. Our objective divine self understands the driving force of our ego with compassion. Healing depends on acceptance and acknowledgment of all parts of our human nature: our multidimensionality, our human ego, and our spiritual self. Accessing unconditional acceptance requires us to allow the objective collective unconscious to influence our subjective nature toward consciousness.

The main principle of healing is our free choice—we make choices that are free of ego-reactive human defensive impulses. Choice is possible when our egos experiences unconditional love and acceptance from our dynamic, objective, creative, integrated, cooperating, multidimensional God-selves.

This objective divine nature in us uses the structure of our personality, with its ego-states, as a vehicle for creative evolution in the material world. Distinguishing between the subjective ego aspects and the objective divine influence in our psyche helps conscious living. We adjust our conditioned beliefs by choice to be more appropriate, based on true life principles. We practice unconditional love and acceptance. We act from our divine center from where we perceive experiences objectively. Our behaviors are liberated from old wounding patterns. We are able to attach, heal, and be happy.

Healing Practices

- Keep a journal.

- Observe and write down your dreams.

- Study your cultural history and observe the themes in the ideas that have influenced you positively and negatively.

- Study your family history and observe the themes in the ideas that have influenced you positively and negatively.

- Study your personal life history. Observe the repeating themes in your behavior and the types of experiences you encounter. Consider how they relate to the themes from your culture and family history.

- Observe your ego-states and identify the ones most active in your everyday life. Talk to them with love and acceptance from the perspective of your God-self while you recognize how they began and why your ego identifies with them. Identify your deepest fears, needs, and defense mechanisms that accompany these ego-states.

- Draw a circle with smaller circles on the periphery to represent all your possible ego-states. Identify them as you become aware of them in your behavior.

- Ask guidance from your God-self.

- Love and accept yourself first and then apply this love and acceptance to all you know.

We swim in an ocean of consciousness. Our bodies occupy the "above" and the "below" as we skim the water surface with powerful strokes toward evolution. We see a colorful rainbow, arching across the heavens, meeting the water, completing its other half-circle beneath the water surface to form a ring of color where our God-self is the center.

Dualism dissipates and the disc completes in wholeness as we illuminate with consciousness. We sense the oceans of the observable and imperceptible simultaneously. We realize that the "pot of gold" is a golden understanding where the end of the rainbow meets at our center—and the visible and the invisible connect.

Appendix: History of South Africa

The times we live in affect our life profoundly. The collective and social history as well as our parents influence who we become. These influences create the nature of our archetypal mother-father-brother-sister experiences. History connects us to our roots and ancestors but also to the seeds of development. As we become aware of self and others as well as the world beyond the personal self, we partake in the evolution of all people.

The "times" that influenced my philosophy and orientation toward healing and growth began with the history of South Africa, my country of birth. This history illustrates the strong unconscious influences on my psyche, which has also been colored by my experience of my family and of society. Thus, one's internal psyche echoes the external world, and the external world mirrors our internal self. Herein lays the challenge to consciousness and growth as we experience life.

The Earliest People

The hunter-gatherer peoples, the San and Khoekhoe, also known as Bushmen and Hottentots or Khoikhoi (Khoisan), occupied South Africa for thousands of years. They occupied the southern and southwestern parts of South Africa. Many hundreds of years before the arrival of the Europeans, the Bantu-speaking people moved into the northeastern and eastern regions of South Africa from the north of Africa. The Thulamela site north of Kruger National Park was first occupied in the thirteenth century. Artifacts from China found in the ruins of Mapungubwe have proved to be the remains of a large twelfth-century trading settlement.

Jan van Riebeeck landed on Cape of Good Hope with ninety men in 1652 under instructions by the Dutch East India Company to build a fort and plant a vegetable garden for the benefit of ships on the Eastern trade route between Europe and India. His relationship with the Khoekhoe was initially one of bartering, but a mutual animosity later developed over cattle theft. The Khoekhoe became suspicious of Van Riebeeck's outpost. This suspicion became a real threat to them in 1657; nine men got land to farm on in South Africa after the release of their contracts with the Dutch. That same year, the first slaves were imported to help work the land. By the time Van Riebeeck left in 1662, 250 people became the first developing white colony in South Africa.

Diseases such as smallpox came with the Europeans, annihilating many of the native people. The Khoekhoe were decimated as an identifiable group. Descendants of some of the Khoisan, slaves from elsewhere in Africa and the East, and white colonists formed the basis of the mixed-race group now known as "colored." It is noteworthy that the slaves from the East brought a potent new ingredient to South Africa's racial and cultural mix, especially with their Islamic religion, recipes, and language.

Governors of the Cape Colony encouraged immigration, and in the early 1700s, independent farmers called "trekboers" began to move into the northern and eastern areas. They encountered Xhosa-speaking people living in the Eastern Cape. Because of territorial threats, uneasy trading relations developed into continuous warfare.

During the second half of the eighteenth century, the Dutch, German, and French Huguenot colonists began to lose their identification with Europe and integrated into a new nation called the Afrikaners.

Britain took the Cape over from the Dutch in 1795. Seven years later, the colony returned to Dutch government—only to become British-ruled again in 1806 because of the alliance between Holland and Napoleon.

The Cape Frontier Wars

In 1820, 5,000 British farming settlers arrived in the eastern frontier to serve as a defensive buffer against the Xhosa, whom the British conflicted with and feared. These settlers later moved to Port Elizabeth and Grahamstown when the land proved difficult to farm. The Xhosa reacted with heroic defiance to protect their independence. They felt threatened with the loss of their land. The Xhosa promised in 1857 to chase the whites into the sea. They slaughtered cattle and destroyed crops. A mass starvation followed.

In 1806, a liberalizing influence arrived in the person of philanthropist missionary, John Philip, friend of the British William Wilberforce, local superintendent of the London Missionary Society.

The Great Trek

The Great Trek started when 12,000 discontented Afrikaner farmers (Boers), who, determined to live independently of British colonial rule, emigrated toward the north and east of South Africa.

During the early decades of the nineteenth century, the great Zulu king, Shaka, raised to power. His wars of conquest and those of Mzilikazi, a general who broke away from Shaka and who wanted to conquer the north, caused a calamitous disruption of the interior known as the "mfecane."

Ironically, these wars caused a great deal of discarded land, and the Trekkers started to use it as farmland, producing food. They believed they were occupying vacant territory, but their claims precipitated more conflict with the Zulu armies.

Many Trekkers moved east into the Natal area, today the province of KwaZulu-Natal, under the leadership of Piet Retief. Shaka's successor murdered Retief and his party of followers and servants while they negotiated for land at the kraal of Dingane.

The Battle of Blood River

A war followed. The Boers won the Battle of Blood River. They began to settle in Natal, but smaller conflicts followed with the British-fearing settlement called Port Natal (later Durban).

Two Boer republics formed on the Highveld, namely the central Orange Free State and South African Republic (Transvaal or Zuid-Afrikaansche Republiek).

By the mid-1800s, the tiny refreshment post at the Cape of Good Hope had grown into an area of white settlement that stretched over virtually all of South Africa.

In some areas, the indigenous Bantu-speaking people maintained their independence, most notably in the northern Natal territories, which were still unmistakably the kingdom of the Zulu. They eventually lost their struggle for independence against white rule, whether British or Boer.

One territory that was to retain independence was the mountain stronghold where King Moshoeshoe had forged the Basotho nation by offering refuge to tribes fleeing the "mfecane." Clashing with the Free Staters, Moshoeshoe asked Britain to annex Basotholand, in 1868. Surrounded by South Africa, known today as Lesotho, has never been a part of it, keeping its independence.

The Cape Colony granted representative legislature in 1853 and self-government in 1872. Between these two dates, the discovery of diamonds in Kimberley introduced a dramatic new element into the economy and, consequently, the political situation.

It became evident that this Subcontinent of South Africa had wealth. Rival claims by the Orange Free State, the Zuid-Afrikaanschee Republiek (ZAR), and Nicholas Waterboer, chief of the West Griquas—a community of mixed race—were defeated, and the area was incorporated into the British Cape Colony in 1880.

A young Cecil John Rhodes, who managed the British territory, was one of many thousands attracted by the diamond diggings that made his fortune. The colony had taken tentative steps toward political equality among the races. The franchise based on non-racial economic qualifications in theory, but it excluded the vast majority of African and colored people in practice. Among those who did qualify, many became politically active across all color lines. The promise of progress toward full political inclusion of the population existed.

Natal and the Battle of Isandhlwana

The Colony of Natal, however, was developing along somewhat different lines. The Zulu nation, assuming threatening proportions, threatened the colonists. Reserves for Zulu refugees operated under traditional African law, but outside of those reserves, British law held sway. All blacks observed the rules of the chiefs in their reserves, but they had no political rights outside their borders.

Natal had an economic advantage due to the cultivation of sugar cane. There was a need to import laborers from India; many—in spite of discrimination—remained in the country after their contracts had expired. They are the forbearers of today's significant and influential Indian population.

The late nineteenth century was an era of aggressive colonial expansion, and the Zulus were bound to come under pressure. However, they did not go down without a fight. Under the rule of King Cetshwayo at Isandhlwana in 1879, they conquered the British army. Nevertheless, their defeat the following year led to the incorporation of Zululand into Natal.

The unpopularity of President T. F. Burgers opened the way for Britain to annex the Transvaal in 1877, but the rebellion and their defeat in the battle of Majuba dealt the British military a blow.

Qualified independence from Britain was achieved in 1881 and full internal autonomy in 1884. The republic elected Afrikaner Paul Kruger as president of the restored but financially strapped people.

The discovery of gold two years later on the Witwatersrand brought a financial turnaround. However, Kruger saw a serious threat to the Afrikaner independence because of huge numbers of newcomers, mostly British, descending on the South African gold fields. The Afrikaners' newfound independence was threatened by incoming foreigners who qualified to vote and change leadership. To counter this threat, he introduced stringent franchise qualification, stipulating that one could achieve residency only after fourteen years.

Rhodes and the Jameson Raid

In the Cape, however, Cecil John Rhodes had become prime minister. The growing discontent of the uitlanders (newcomers) and the exasperation of the mining magnates in the ZAR served his overriding vision of a federation of British-controlled states in Southern Africa. Rhodes's first attempt at takeover came to a humiliating end when he botched a plan to suppress an uitlander "upraising." Leander Starr Jameson was under orders to lead a raid into Johannesburg. The upraising did not happen; Jameson rode precipitously into the Transvaal and had to surrender. Rhodes resigned.

The Jameson Raid had a polarizing effect. Afrikaners in the Cape and the Orange Free State, though disapproving of Kruger in many ways, became more sympathetic to his anti-British stance. The Orange Free State, under President M. T. Steyn, formed a military alliance with the Transvaal.

The Anglo-Boer War

In Britain, however, Rhodes and Jameson were popular heroes. It kept pressure on Kruger, and the Anglo-Boer South African War began in October 1899. Half a million British soldiers squared up against some 65,000 Boers. The conflict between the Boers and the British pulled black South Africans into it from both sides.

Britain's military reputation suffered a blow as the Boers set siege to Ladysmith, Kimberley, and Mafiking. Under Major General Herbert Kitchener and Field Marshal Sir Frederick Sleigh Roberts, the British offensive gained force and occupied Bloemfontein, Johannesburg, and Pretoria by 1900. Kruger fled for Europe.

The Boers intensified their guerrilla war. General Jan Smuts, who had been Kruger's state attorney, led his troops to within 190 kilometers of Cape Town, and Kitchener adopted a scorched-earth policy in British retaliation that set up racially separate civilian concentration camps in which some 26,000 Boer women and children and 14,000 black and colored people died in appalling conditions.

The war ended in Boer defeat at the Peace of Vereeniging in 1902. Many blacks saw the British victory as an opportunity to put all four colonies on an equal and just footing, but the treaty left their franchise rights yet again in the hands of white authorities. The ex-Boer republics retained the whites-only franchise.

In 1909, a delegation appointed by the South African Native Convention, including representatives of the colored and Indian populations, went to London to plead the case of the country's black population. When the Union of South Africa came into being on May 31, 1910, the only province with a non-racial franchise was the Cape. Black people could not become members of parliament. Of the estimated 6,000,000 inhabitants of the Union in that year, 67 percent were black African, 9 percent were colored, and 2.5 percent were Asian.

The South African Party, a merging of the previous Afrikaner parties, held power under the premiership of General Louis Botha.

The 1913 Land Act and the ANC

The Masters and Servants Act, the reservation of skilled work for whites, the pass laws, the Native Poll Tax, and the 1913 Land Act reserving 90 percent of the country for white ownership were all repressive measures to entrench white power.

The African National Congress (ANC) formed on January 8, 1912, in Bloemfontein. The committee included Sol Plaatje (a young black diarist from Mafiking) as secretary; the first president of the ANC was Rev. John L. Dube. Both formed part of a second unsuccessful delegation to London—this time to protest the land grab.

Resistance started to assume a more outspoken and militant form. Several hundred black women marched in Bloemfontein to protest against the use of passes every month. Arrests followed participants in other similar protests in other places. Jail treated the women especially harshly.

Mohandas Gandhi

The Indian community also suffered vicious racist treatment. In 1891, the Orange Free State expelled them. Mohandas Gandhi, then a young lawyer, arrived in South Africa in 1892. He became a leader of the Indian resistance. The struggle against the £3 Indian poll tax in Natal involved a mass strike in which a number of Indians died. Exemption of this tax occurred in 1914, when Gandhi, known as Mahatma, left the country.

Afrikaner Polarization

In the white camp, Botha and Smuts were in favor of reconciliation with English South Africans, but they did not represent the whole of the embittered Afrikaner nation, who still resented the atrocities against women and children during the Boer War. J. B. M. Hertzog formed a conservative Nationalist Party. Afrikaners showed polarized sentiments when South Africa entered the First World War in support of Britain. Anti-British Afrikaners unsuccessfully rebelled against this support. The ANC supported involvement in the war, hoping to gain support back from the British government. An unknown number of black soldiers died in this war.

South Africa gained control over the previously German-held South West Africa—now Namibia—because of the war; the territory became a Union mandate.

Black Workers, White Workers

Inspired by the October Revolution in Russia, action strikes marked the post-war period. In 1918, a million black mine workers went on strike for higher wages, and 71,000 did the same in 1920. The latter strike was successful in negotiating a wage increase. Between these strikes, 1919 saw the formation of the Industrial and Commercial Workers' Union of South Africa and the convening of the South African Indian Congress. In the same year, Botha died and Smuts became Prime Minister.

Official (white) South Africa was taking its place in the wider world because of the First World War, and the ANC was beginning to see itself as part of the wider African efforts against colonialism in Africa. In its 1918 Constitution, it referred to itself as a "Pan African Association", and the organization attended the second congress of the international Pan African Movement in 1921 (not to be confused with the later South African Pan-Africanist Congress).

Another miners' strike was looming. Rising costs and a falling gold price led the Chamber of Mines to allow the lower-paid African miners to do semi-skilled work. White miners reacted violently in a 1922 strike, but Smuts suppressed them militantly. Hertzog's Nationalists found increased support in the white Labour Party, and an election pact saw Smuts ousted and Hertzog made Prime Minister in 1924.

The next decade saw Hertzog successfully working for increased independence from British control and greater job reservation security for whites. Franchise acts extended the vote to all white men and women, but left the still-existing black vote in the Cape restricted to men.

Birth of the Nationalist Party

The government's popularity with its voters declined, however, with economic depression in the early 1930s, forcing Hertzog into a Smuts coalition government in 1933 (the year before South Africa became independent from Great Britain). Their parties fused as the United Party, but Hertzog's move balanced D. F. Malan's breaking away to the right with his new Nationalist Party as a political home for the extreme Afrikaner nationalists.

In 1936, the common roll removed black Cape voters. Laws passed that halted black urbanization and compelled municipalities to segregate black African and white residents.

The Hertzog-Smuts coalition fell apart with the Second World War; Smuts won the battle to form a government that took South Africa into the war. Afrikaner opposition to the war strengthened support for Malan.

ANC Youth League, Natal Indian Congress

At the same time, developments in the ANC marked the beginning of fifty years of conflict with the Nationalist Party. The ANC Youth League formed in April 1944. Its first president was A. M. Lembede, but he died three years later. Nelson Mandela was secretary during that time. Oliver Tambo and Walter Sisulu had important influences on the Youth League in the broader ANC.

Rapid industrial expansion existed during that time, but whites still got the skilled work. Black resistance was strengthened by the black influx into urban areas. These people experienced continuous repression. Smuts introduced a bill aimed at curtailing the movement of Indian residence and property ownership in 1946, but this led to mass defiance and the rapid expansion of the Natal Indian Congress.

Apartheid Entrenched

The ideals of the United Nations cast a spotlight on the country's racial inequity, and the first of many attacks on the country in the General Assembly came from the Indian government in 1946.

The Nationalist Party was gathering strength, however, and in a surprise result, gained power in the 1948 election. Apartheid became official government ideology, a power that relinquished only in 1994. The 1950s were to bring increasingly repressive laws against black South Africans. The obvious consequence was increased resistance.

The Group Areas Act created a rigid division of land along racial lines. The Population Registration Act of 1950 classified all citizens by race. The Pass Laws of 1952 restricted black people's movement. The Separate Amenities Act of 1953 introduced petty apartheid—a string of prohibitive legislation—for example, the separation of people of color on buses and in post offices. In that year, Malan retired and J. G. Strijdom became prime minister.

The Defiance Campaign

The mass mobilization of the Defiance Campaign was a reaction to all the conflict in 1952. Despite non-violent principles, their resistance led to the jailing of thousands of participants. Resistance groups united to form the Congress Alliance, which included black, colored, Indian, and white organizations, as well as the South African Congress of Trade Unions.

In 1954, a campaign launched ideas to improve the inferior Bantu Education System.

The Freedom Charter

South Africa's racial injustices were resolved reasonably peacefully in the 1950s. However, apartheid transmuted itself into the policy of separate development: the division of the black population into ethnic nations, each of which was to have its own "homeland" and eventual "independence."

Two of the most significant events of the decade occurred in 1955. Unable to gain the two-thirds majority required by the 1910 Constitution to remove coloreds from the common voters' roll, the government changed the composition of the Senate by increasing its size (and consequently its Nationalist majority) to give it the required majority in a joint sitting of the Senate and the House of Assembly. The second event was a watershed moment.

An ANC campaign gathered mass input on freedom demands to draft the Freedom Charter, based on the principles of human rights and non-racialism. The Congress of the People in Soweto signed this charter on June 26, 1955. As a result, 156 leaders of the ANC and its allies were charged with high treason in 1956. The longest trial in South African history resulted in the acquittal of all accused in 1961.

H. F. Verwoerd succeeded Strijdom who died in 1958. The following year, both the houses of parliament and the Cape Provincial Council removed black African representatives. On the other side of the political fence, the Pan-Africanist Congress (PAC), founded by Robert Sobukwe, broke away from the Congress Alliance. Polarization heightened in the 1960s.

The Sharpeville Massacre

A turning point came on March 21, 1960, in Sharpeville, when a PAC-organized passive anti-pass campaign came to a bloody conclusion with police killing sixty-nine unarmed protesters. A state of emergency introduced detention without trial, and the ANC, the PAC, and other organizations were declared illegal. Resistance groups went underground.

South Africa's isolation increased in 1961 when, following a white referendum, South Africa became a republic, and Verwoerd separated South Africa from the Commonwealth.

The group Umkhonto we Sizwe (The Spear of the Nation) emerged with acts of sabotage against the government at the end of 1961. Originally formed by a group of individuals within the ANC, including Nelson Mandela, this group became their organization's armed wing.

A new stage of international pressure began when the UN General Assembly called on its members to institute economic sanctions against South Africa. Mandela, in the meantime, had traveled through Africa, making contact with numerous leaders. Going underground on his return, he was arrested in Natal in August 1962 and received a three-year sentence for incitement.

The Rivonia Trial

In July 1963, a police raid on the Rivonia farm Lilliesleaf led to the arrest of several of Mandela's senior ANC colleagues, including Walter Sisulu. Mandela and the others stood trial on sabotage. They all were sentenced to life imprisonment in 1964 and taken to Robben Island.

In September 1966, B. J. Vorster became prime minister after the assassination of Verwoerd in Parliament. Segregation was even more strictly enforced. Reeling under the blow of the Rivonia Trial, the ANC nevertheless continued to operate, regrouping at the Morogoro Conference in Tanzania in 1969.

The first half of the next decade marked increasing repression, increasing militancy in the resistance camp, and extensive strikes.

June 16, 1976

The decisive moment came on June 16, 1976, when Soweto students marched against being taught in Afrikaans, the language they considered that of the oppressor. Police fired on them, precipitating a massive flood of violence that overwhelmed the country.

Transkei was first to accept nominal independence in 1976 after the promotion of a "homeland" policy.

A new movement, known as Black Consciousness, became increasingly influential. The death of its charismatic founder, Steve Biko, because of police brutality, shocked the world in 1977.

P. W. Botha, who became prime minister in 1978 after Vorster's retirement, tried to co-opt the colored and Indian population in the early 1980s with a new Constitution establishing a Tricameral Parliament with separate houses for these groups. The Constitution also did away with the post of prime minister and provided for an executive state president. Opposition came from both left and right. A section of the right wing split off from the National Party. The United Democratic Front, an internal coalition of anti-apartheid groups, organized highly successful boycotts of the colored and Indian elections in 1984.

State of Emergency

There was a further escalation of violence, with the country being governed—as far as it was governable—under a state of emergency in a spiral of revolution and repression. International sanctions increased. Among the other organizations in the spotlight at this time were the trade union body Cosatu and Chief Mangosuthu Buthelezi's Inkatha; the latter was involved in bloody conflict with pro-ANC factions.

In 1989, the logjam started to break up. Mandela and P. W. Botha entered secret negotiations. Dissension within the Nationalist Party, in combination with Botha's ill health, led to his resignation, and F. W. de Klerk replaced him. History was about to change.

After an election in September 1989, de Klerk released Walter Sisulu and seven other political prisoners.

On February 2, 1990, F. W. de Klerk lifted restrictions on thirty-three opposition groups, including the ANC, the PAC, and the Communist

Party, at the opening of Parliament. The release of Mandela happened on February 11 after twenty-seven years in prison.

The piecemeal dismantling of restrictive legislation began. Political groups started negotiating the ending of white minority rule, and in early 1992, the white electorate endorsed De Klerk's stance on these negotiations in a referendum.

However, violence continued unabated; a massacre at the township of Boipatong caused the ANC to withdraw temporarily from constitutional talks. However, in 1993, the Government of National Unity reached an agreement that allowed a partnership of the old regime and the new. The negotiations generated optimism, but the assassination of Chris Hani, the secretary-general of the Communist Party, shattered the ideal. Only a prompt appeal to the nation by Mandela averted a massive reaction. At the end of 1993, twenty-one political parties agreed to an interim Constitution.

First Democratic Elections

On April 26, 27, and 28, 1994, South Africa held its first democratic election with victory to the ANC in an alliance with the Communist Party and Cosatu. Nelson Mandela became president on May 10, with F. W. de Klerk and the ANC's Thabo Mbeki as deputy presidents. Mandela's presidency successful negotiated a new Constitution. A massive restructuring of the civil service and redirecting of the national priorities to address the results of apartheid began. The Truth and Reconciliation Commission was set up to investigate the wrongs of the past.

In the country's second democratic election on June 2, 1999, the ANC marginally increased its majority, and Thabo Mbeki became president. The New Nationalist Party lost ground and gave up their position to the Democratic Party, which later became the Democratic Alliance.

In 2004, South Africa's third democratic election went off peacefully; Thabo Mbeki and the ANC returned to power, and the Democratic Alliance retained its position as official opposition.

Bibliography

Assagioli, Roberto. *Psychosynthesis: A Collection of Basic Writings.* Penguin Books, 1976.

——. *Transpersonal Development: The Dimension Beyond Psychosynthesis.* Milton Keynes, UK: Lightning Source Publishers, 2007.

Bateson, Gregory. *Mind and Nature: A Necessary Unity.* Bantam Books, 1980.

Berne, Eric. *Games People Play: The Psychology of Human Relationships. The Basic Handbook of Transactional Analysis.* Ballantine Books, 1996.

Bloch, Jayni. "Liberation from Unconscious Repetitive Conflict-Cycles, using Healing Indicators from Archtypal Themes." *Eight Energy Psychology Conference.* Toronto: Energy Psychology Conference, 2006.

——. "The Light Bulb Experince: The Rational Link in Metaphor." *Canadian Psychological Association Annual Conference.* Quebec City: Canadian Psychological Association Annual Conference, 2001.

—. "The 'Next Step" in the Evolution of Relationships; a Quantum Leap to New Meaning and Healing of Union." *Ninth Annual Energy Psychology Conference*. Toronto: Ninth Annual Energy Psychology Conference, 2007.

—. "The Relationship between Spiritual-Psychological Life-Challenges and Archetyped indicates and mobilizes the Healing Process." *International Conference on Spirituality and Mental Health (4th)*. Saint Paul University, Ottawa: 4th International Conference on Spirituality and Mental Health, 2009.

—. "The Subconscious Mind, Resource in the Therapy Process." *The Canadian Psychological Association Annual Conference*. Ottawa: The Canadian Psychological Association Annual Conference, 2000.

—. "Transformation: Moving out of the Box." *International Milton Erickson Foundation Conference*. Phoenix, AZ: Milton Erickson Foundation Conference , 2004.

Callahan, Roger. *Tapping the Healer Within: Using Thought-Field Therapy to Instantly Conquer Your Fears, Anxieties and Emotional Distress*. Contemporary Books, 2001.

Capra, Fritjof. *The Tao of Physics: An Exploration of the Parallels between Modern Physics and Eastern Mysticism. Berkley*, California: Shambhala Publications, 1975.

—. *Uncommon Wisdom: Conversations with Remarkable People*. Simon & Schuster, 1988.

Dethlefsen, Thorward and Dahlke, Rudiger, and Peter translated by Lemesurier. *The Healing Power of Illness: The Meaning of Symptoms and How to Interpret them*. Massachusetts: Element Books, 1991.

Edinger, Edward, F. *Ego and Archetype.* C. G. Jung Foundation Book, 1972.

Edinger, Edward, F. *Ego and Archetype: Individuation and the Religious Function of the Psyche.* Boston and London: Shambhala, 1992.

Erickson, Milton.H. *Healing In Hypnosis. Volume 1.* New York: Irvington Publishers, Inc, 1092.

Estes, Clarissa Pinkola. *Women Who Run with the Wolves: Contacting the Power of the Wild Woman.* UK: Rider, 1992.

Feinstein, David, and Donna, and Graig, Gary Eden. *The Promise of Energy Psychology: Revolutionary Tools for Dramatic Personal Change.* USA: Penguin Group Inc., 2005.

Green, Liz, and Sasportas, Howard. *Dynamics of the Unconscious: Seminars in Psychological Astrology, Volume 1 and Volume 2.* Maine: Samuel Wiser Inc., 1989.

Harris, Bud. *The Father Quest: Rediscovering an Elemental Psychic Force.* Alexander, North Carolina: Alexander Books, 1996.

Harris, Thomas. *I'm OK, You're OK.* Harper and Row Publishers, 1996.

Hawkind, David. *Power versus Force: The Hidden Determinants of Human Behavior.* Hay House Inc., 2002.

Hawkins, David. *Discovery of the Presence of God: Devotional Nonduality.* Veritas Publishing, 2007.

—. *Pragmatism and the Meaning of Truth.* Harvard University Press, 2005.

Heuer, Gottfried. *Sacral Revolutions: Reflection on the Work of Andrew Samuels: Cutting Edges in Psychoanalysis and Jungian Analysis.* New York, NY: Routledge Taylor & Francis Group, 2010.

Hillman, James. *Blue Fire.* Harper Perennial, 1991.

James, William. *The Soul's Code: In Search of Character and Calling.* New York: Warner Books with Random House, 1996.

Johnson, Robert, A. *The Psychology of Romantic Love.* London: Arkana, 1983.

—. *Transformation: Understanding the Three Levels of Masculine Consciousness.* Harper Collins, 1991.

Johnson, Susan, M. *Emotionally Focused Couple Therapy with Trauma Survivors: Strengthening Attachment Bonds.* New York: The Guilford Press, 2002.

Johnson, Susan, M., and Whiffen, Valerie, E. *Attachment Processes in Couple and Family Therapy.* New York: The Guilford Press, 2003.

Johnson. Robert, A. *Inner Work: Using Dreams and Active Imagination for Personal Growth.* Harper Collins Publishers, 1986.

Jung, Carl, Gustav. *Archetypes and the Collective Unconscious (Collective works of C.G. Jung. Volume 9, Part 1.* Princeton University Press, 1981, Second Edition.

—. *Aspects of the Feminine,* Translated by Hull, R. F. C. Ark Paperbacks, Bollingen Foundation, 1986.

—. *The Psycholgy of the Transference,* Translated by Hull, R. F. C. Ark Paperbacks, Bollingen Foundation, 1966.

Lankton, Stephen R., and Carol H. Lankton. *The Answer within: A Clinical Framework of Ericksonian Hypnotherapy.* New York: Brunner/Mazel Publishers, 1983.

Lowinsky, Naomi, Ruth. *The Motherline: Every Woman's Journey to Find her Female Roots.* Fisher King Press, 1992.

Lundsted, Betty. *Astrological Insights into Personality.* California: Astro Computing Services, 1980.

Mann, A. T. *The Divine Plot: Astrology and Reincarnation.* Element Books, 1991.

—. *The Round Art: The Astrology of Time and Space.* Paper Tiger, A Dragon's World Limited Imprint, 1979.

Nesfield-Cookson, Bernard. *Rudolf Steiner's Vision of Love: Spiritual Science and the Logic of the Heart.* Wellingborough, Northamptonshire, England: The Aquarian Press, Thoorsons Publishing Group, 1989.

Padesky, Christine A. and Greenberge, Dennis. *Clinician's Guide to Mind over Mood.* New York: The Guilford Press, 1995.

Perls, Frederick, S., Ralph, F. Hefferline, and Paul Goodman. *Gestalt Therapy: Excitement and Growth in the Human Personality.* England: Penguin Books Ltd., 1976.

Perls, Friedrich, Saloman. *Gestalt Approach and Eye Witness to Therapy.* Hushion House, 1973.

Phillips, Maggie and Frederick, Claire. *Healing the Divided Self: Clinical and Ericksonian Hypnotherapy* for *Dissociative Conditions*. New York: W.W. Norton and Company, 1995.

Rogers, Carl. *Client-Centered Therapy: Its Current Practice, Implications and Theory*. London: Constable, 1951.

Rohr, Richard. *The Naked Now: Learning to See as the Mystics See*. New York: The Crossroad Publishing Company, 2000.

Rohr, Richard, with Martos, Joseph. *From Wild Man to Wise Man: Reflections on Male Spirituality*. Cincinnati, Ohio: St. Anthony Messenger Press, 2005.

Rossi, Ernest Lawrence. *The Breakout Heuristic: The New Neuroscience of Mirror Neurons, Consciousness and Creativity in Human Relationships*. Phoenix, Arizona: The Milton H. Erickson Foundation Press, 2007.

Stone, Barbara. *Invisible Roots: How Healing Past Life Trauma Can Liberate Your Present*. Santa Rosa, CA: Energy Psychology Press, 2008.

Tapas, Fleming. "Tapas Acupressure Technique Workshop: TAT." *Energy Psychology Conference*. Toronto: Energy Psychology Conference, 2005.

Tarnas, Richard. *The Passion of the Western Mind: Understanding the Ideas That Have Shaped Our World View*. New York: A Ballantine Book, The Random Publishing Group, 1991.

Taylor, Jill, Bolte. *My Stroke of Insight: A Brain Scientist's Personal Journey*; 1st Edition. Plume, 2009.

Valentine, Christine. *Images of the Psyche: Exploring the Planets through Psychology and Myth.* Great Britain: Element Books, 1991.

Von Franz, Marie-Louise. *Alchemical Active Imagination.* Boston and London: Shambhala, 1997.

Watkins, John, G. and Watkins, Helen, H. *Hypnotherapeutic Techniques: The Practice of Clinical Hypnosis, Volume 1 and Volume 2.* New York: Irvington Publishers, Inc., 1987 and 1992.

Zeig, Jeffrey, K and Gilligan, Stephen, G. *Brief Therapy: Myths, Methods, and Metaphors.* New York: Brunner / Mazel Publishers, 1990.

www.southafrica.info – A brief history of South Africa

CPSIA information can be obtained at www.ICGtesting.com
Printed in the USA
LVOW101242251112

308724LV00004B/491/P